NEPHROLOGY RESEARCH AND CLINICAL DEVELOPMENTS

ACUTE KIDNEY INJURY: CAUSES, DIAGNOSIS, AND TREATMENT

Nephrology Research and Clinical Developments

Additional books in this series can be found on Nova's website under the Series tab.

Additional E-books in this series can be found on Nova's website under the E-books tab.

NEPHROLOGY RESEARCH AND CLINICAL DEVELOPMENTS

ACUTE KIDNEY INJURY: CAUSES, DIAGNOSIS, AND TREATMENT

JONATHAN D. MENDOZA

EDITOR

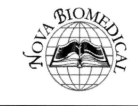

Nova Science Publishers, Inc.

New York

For permission to use material from this book please contact us:
Telephone 631-231-7269; Fax 631-231-8175
Web Site: http://www.novapublishers.com

NOTICE TO THE READER

The Publisher has taken reasonable care in the preparation of this book, but makes no expressed or implied warranty of any kind and assumes no responsibility for any errors or omissions. No liability is assumed for incidental or consequential damages in connection with or arising out of information contained in this book. The Publisher shall not be liable for any special, consequential, or exemplary damages resulting, in whole or in part, from the readers' use of, or reliance upon, this material. Any parts of this book based on government reports are so indicated and copyright is claimed for those parts to the extent applicable to compilations of such works.

Independent verification should be sought for any data, advice or recommendations contained in this book. In addition, no responsibility is assumed by the publisher for any injury and/or damage to persons or property arising from any methods, products, instructions, ideas or otherwise contained in this publication.

This publication is designed to provide accurate and authoritative information with regard to the subject matter covered herein. It is sold with the clear understanding that the Publisher is not engaged in rendering legal or any other professional services. If legal or any other expert assistance is required, the services of a competent person should be sought. FROM A DECLARATION OF PARTICIPANTS JOINTLY ADOPTED BY A COMMITTEE OF THE AMERICAN BAR ASSOCIATION AND A COMMITTEE OF PUBLISHERS.

Additional color graphics may be available in the e-book version of this book.

LIBRARY OF CONGRESS CATALOGING-IN-PUBLICATION DATA

Acute kidney injury : causes, diagnosis, and treatments / editor, Jonathan
D. Mendoza.
  p. ; cm.
  Includes bibliographical references and index.
  ISBN 978-1-61209-790-9 (hardcover : alk. paper)
  1. Acute renal failure. I. Mendoza, Jonathan D.
  [DNLM: 1. Acute Kidney Injury. WJ 342]
  RC918.R4A328 2011
  616.6'14--dc22
2011002412

Published by Nova Science Publishers, Inc. † New York

Contents

Short Communication

Preface

Acute kidney injury (AKI) is a common condition with significant associated morbidity and mortality. Although impressive progress has been made in the understanding of the molecular and biochemical mechanisms of kidney injury, as well as in the clinical care of patients with AKI, outcomes have remained disturbingly static over the last 40-50 years. This new book presents topical research data in the study of the causes, diagnosis and treatment of acute kidney injury. Topics discussed include classification of AKI; acute renal failure in the newborn; kidney ischemia and reperfusion injury; pandemic H1N1 influenza A infection and AKI; the role of oxidative stress in renal ischemia; biomarkers in acute kidney injury and B2 adrenoceptor therapy in AKI.

Chapter 1 – Over the last decades, more than 35 different definitions have been used to define acute kidney injury (AKI). Multiple definitions for AKI have obviously led to a great disparity in the reported incidence of AKI making it difficult or even impossible to compare the various published studies focusing on AKI. For example, according to the definition employed, the previously described incidence of AKI in the critically ill patients has varied between 1 and 25 percent and mortality has ranged from 15 to 60%. In May 2004, a new classification, the "Risk Injury Failure Loss of Kidney Function End-stage" kidney disease (RIFLE) classification, has been proposed in order to define and stratify the severity of AKI. This system relies on changes in serum creatinine or glomerular filtration rate and/or urine output, and it has been largely demonstrated that RIFLE criteria allow the identification of a significant proportion of hospitalized patients in numerous settings as having AKI, permit to monitoring AKI severity and predict well patients'outcome. More recently, in March 2007, a modified version of the RIFLE, the Acute Kidney Injury Network (AKIN) classification has been proposed in order to increase the sensitivity and specificity of AKI diagnosis. Until the present, however, the benefit of those modifications in the clinical practice has not been clearly demonstrated. In this chapter we describe the AKI definition and staging according to the RIFLE and AKIN classifications, focusing on their main differences, advantages and limitations. We also review the more relevant studies validating such classifications in different settings of hospitalized patients.

Chapter 2 – Despite advances in neonatal and perinatal medicine the assessment of the renal function of newborns remains a major challenge. The unique features of neonates defy the ability to understand and define acute kidney injury (AKI) in this age group. The studies on the subject are scarce and mostly based on a small numbers of patients and performed in single centers. Up until now, observational studies suggest that critically ill neonates have high rates of AKI with a guarded prognosis. Moreover, newborns with AKI can develop a renal function impairment, proteinuria and hypertension requiring long term monitoring. Appropriate evaluation of renal function represents the first step towards the recognition and early treatment of AKI (elimination of risk factors) and a change in the short and long-term prognosis of critically ill newborns.

Chapter 3 – Acute kidney injury (AKI) is an important occurrence characterized by a sudden decrease in renal function. Acute kidney injury (AKI) caused by ischemia and reperfusion injury (IRI) is a common clinical syndrome, associated with high morbidity and mortality. Much of the increased risk of death associated with AKI is from non-renal complications, usually related to multi-organ dysfunction.

Serum creatinine which has been considered the main diagnostic test for AKI rises late in the pathophysiology and is an inaccurate marker of acute changes in glomerular filtration rate. New biomarkers are in evaluation with the aim to identify a possible AKI before oliguria or elevated serum creatinine is detectable, as those criteria already reflect established renal tubular cell injury. Toll-like receptors (TLR), neutrophil gelatinase-associated lipocalin (NGAL), liver-type fatty acid binding protein (L-FABP) or kidney injury molecule-1 (KIM-1) which levels increase prior to the serum creatinine elevation are promising and have been used in clinical trials.

In kidney transplantation the occurrence of ischemia and reperfusion injury (IRI) can delay graft function with the need of postoperative dialysis. Also IRI has been associated with chronic allograft rejection and has influence on long-term graft survival. Our group showed recently that as early as 24 hours after kidney ischemia and reperfusion injury in mice a significant increase of TLR2 and TLR4 expression occurs not only on resident cells but also in kidney infiltrating cells (leukocytes). The increase in these markers was associated with the decrease of kidney function (as depicted by the increase in serum creatinine and urea levels) and acute tubular necrosis. The use of an immunomodulatory agent (FTY720) decreased TLR levels and provided earlier recovery of renal function with no effect on kidney structure. These data suggest that studies for the discovery of new biomarkers with early expression and the restriction of inflammatory responses are promising tools for diagnosis and therapies to reduce acute kidney injury.

Chapter 4 – Several studies have found that post-angiographic acute kidney injury (AKI) is a risk of long-term mortality after coronary angiography. These studies have also found that acute hemodynamic disturbances requiring hemodynamic support have a strong impact both on the incidence of AKI and on the prognosis after coronary angiography.

The impact of AKI on prognosis might have been affected by hemodynamic factors in these studies because hemodynamic instability in itself is, not only closely related to the incidence of post-angiographic AKI, but also a strong risk factor for the prognosis. Therefore, we aimed to study the impact of AKI on long-term prognosis after coronary angiography among hospital survivors in relation with hemodynamic variables.

We found that AKI is a predictor of long-term prognosis in the whole studied population, however, its impact was attenuated among hemodynamically stable patients. This result suggested that the impact of AKI for the hemodynamically stable patients was attenuated from the overall patients.

As seen in this study, the cause of AKI in itself could affect the long-term prognosis after AKI. In order to evaluate the long-term prognosis of AKI patients, clinicians need to take the cause of AKI into consideration.

Chapter 5 – Acute kidney injury (AKI) is a serious complication of cardiac surgery. Cardiac surgery-associated AKI (CSA-AKI) is associated with high in-hospital mortality, complicated hospital course, a high risk of infectious complications and high utilization of resources. The spectrum of CSA-AKI can range from subclinical renal injury to severe AKI requiring Renal Replacement Therapy (RRT). Patients with AKI requiring RRT have 30-day mortality rates in excess of 40%. Despite the advances in bypass techniques, intensive care, and delivery of RRT, mortality and morbidity associated with AKI have not changed much in recent years. Even small increases in serum creatinine (SCr) after surgery, that is not associated with need for RRT, are also associated with significantly increased risk of mortality, both in the short and long-term. The normalization of elevated serum creatinine prior to discharge from the hospital does not appear to reduce the risk of increased mortality in these patients. There is however, considerable heterogeneity in the mortality rates in different studies due to the lack of uniform criteria for the definition of AKI. Herein we discuss the proposed pathomechanisms of CSA-AKI and recent strategies for diagnosis and prevention of CSA-AKI.

Chapter 6 – Acute kidney injury (AKI) is the main cause of acute renal failure (ARF) in native kidneys, being associated with a high mortality and loss of kidney function in the long term. There are considerable data implicating the important role of the innate and adaptive immune response in AKI. Toll-like receptor (TLR) are the best-characterized receptors of innate immunity, able to recognize pathogens associated molecular patterns (PAMPs), such as LPS, beginning an inflammatory response and also shaping the adaptive immunity. Endogenous ligands released from damaged or stressed tissues seem to signal through TLRs. In addition, TLR can activate dendritic cells (DCs). Upon activation, DCs induce naive T cells to proliferate and polarize to differentiate T helper subtypes. Recently, another innate immune response receptor, the Nod-like receptors (NLR), was identified. The role of the NLR in kidney pathologies is less clear but evidence of its involvement in renal diseases has been reported. Besides, the involvement of innate immune cells, T cells are also incriminated in the pathogenesis of AKI. Specifically, CD4+ Th1 cells seem to be the most detrimental. The mechanism of action of these cells is still on debate; although it seems to involve an antigen-independent activation. In this review, we will discuss the significance of the innate and adaptive immune receptors in the development of AKI secondary to different insults such as ischemia and sepsis.

Chapter 7 – The recent global outbreak of pandemic H1N1 (pH1N1) influenza A infection strained global intensive care unit resources as critically ill patients often required respiratory support. Early data suggests a large proportion of patients suffered acute kidney injury and required renal replacement therapy. This review will outline the impact of the pH1N1 outbreak, discuss the epidemiology and mechanisms of acute kidney injury due to pH1N1, and suggest general treatment recommendations.

Chapter 8 - Acute kidney injury (AKI) is a common condition with significant associated morbidity and mortality. Although impressive progress has been made in the understanding of the molecular and biochemical mechanisms of kidney injury as well as in the clinical care of patients with AKI, outcomes have remained disturbingly static over the last 40 – 50 years. Reliance on current measures of renal dysfunction, such as serum creatinine and blood urea nitrogen, has contributed to the slow translation of basic science discovery to therapeutically effective approaches in clinical practice. Insensitivity of commonly used biomarkers of renal dysfunction not only prevents timely diagnosis and estimation of injury severity, but also delays administration of putative therapeutic agents. A number of serum and urinary proteins have been identified that may herald AKI prior to a rise in serum creatinine. Further characterization of these candidate biomarkers will clarify their utility and define new diagnostic and prognostic paradigms for AKI, facilitate clinical trials and lead to novel effective therapies. Thus, we are positioned to soon have clinically useful biomarkers which, either alone or in combination, will facilitate earlier diagnosis, earlier targeted intervention, and improved outcomes.

Chapter 9 - Endotoxemia caused by Gram-negative bacteria can result in sepsis and organ dysfunction, which includes kidney injury and renal failure. The renal β_2-adrenoceptor (β_2-AR) system has an anti-inflammatory influence on the cytokine network during the course of immunologic responses. The previous reports indicated that the administration of β_2-AR agonists was found to attenuate the stimulation of renal TNF-α associated with lipopolysaccharide and Shiga toxin-2 of hemolytic uremic syndrome (HUS), which is considered to be a central mediator of the pathophysiologic changes. On the other hand, an altered expression and/or function of β_2-AR have been considered to be a pathogenetic factor in some disease states with inflammation; for example, heart failure and renal failure. These observations would suggest that blockade of functional β_2-AR activation might be associated with an increase risk for organ dysfunction following severe sepsis. In this chapter, we reviewed sepsis-induced renal injury and the genomic information to identify groups of patients with a high risk of developing sepsis-induced acute renal failure. In addition, we attempt to demonstrate a new insight into the immunological importance of β_2-AR activation in sepsis and an application of β_2-AR to septic renal failure and HUS. Furthermore, an *in vivo* β_2-AR gene therapy for the replacement of lost receptors as a consequence of sepsis was also described.

Short Communication - Acute kidney injury (AKI) occurs frequently in various clinical contexts. There is increasing evidence that AKI directly contributes to dysfunction in the lung, brain, liver, heart, and other organs. Various drugs have been developed and are now being used clinically, but with limited success. AKI continues to contribute significantly to morbidity and mortality in the intensive care unit (ICU) setting, especially when associated with distant organ dysfunction. Recently, many studies have examined the mechanisms underlying AKI. In particular, the role of reactive oxygen species (ROS) in AKI pathogenesis has received much attention. ROS include hydroxyl radicals that react with nearby tissues, proteins, enzymes, cell membranes, and DNA. Hydroxyl radicals themselves are short-lived, but they damage biomolecules, affecting cellular and tissue function. The key location for ROS generation is the mitochondrion. Excessive ROS generation damages the mitochondria themselves, leading to cellular dysfunction and apoptosis. Anti-oxidants are involved in regulating intracellular ROS levels and are generally thought to attenuate oxidative stress, cellular and tissue injury, and mitochondrial damage. These findings collectively point to ROS as important targets for AKI treatment.

In: Acute Kidney Injury: Causes, Diagnosis and Treatments   ISBN: 978-1-61209-790-9
Editor: Jonathan D. Mendoza, pp. 1-18   © 2011 Nova Science Publishers, Inc.

Chapter I

How to Define and Classify Acute Kidney Injury (AKI): The "Risk Injury Failure Loss of Kidney Function End-Stage Kidney Disease" (RIFLE) and "Acute Kidney Injury Network" (AKIN) Classifications

José António Lopes [*] *and Sofia Jorge*
Faculty of Medicine of Lisbon, Department of Nephrology and Renal Transplantation
Hospital de Santa Maria, Av. Prof. Egas Moniz, 1649-035, Lisbon, Portugal

Abstract

Over the last decades, more than 35 different definitions have been used to define acute kidney injury (AKI). Multiple definitions for AKI have obviously led to a great disparity in the reported incidence of AKI making it difficult or even impossible to compare the various published studies focusing on AKI. For example, according to the definition employed, the previously described incidence of AKI in the critically ill patients has varied between 1 and 25 percent and mortality has ranged from 15 to 60%. In May 2004, a new classification, the Risk Injury Failure Loss of kidney function End-stage kidney disease (RIFLE) classification, has been proposed in order to define and stratify the severity of AKI. This system relies on changes in serum creatinine or glomerular filtration rate and/or urine output, and it has been largely demonstrated that RIFLE criteria allow the identification of a significant proportion of hospitalized patients in numerous settings as having AKI, permit to monitoring AKI severity and predict well patients'outcome. More recently, in March 2007, , a modified version of the RIFLE, the Acute Kidney Injury Network (AKIN) classification has been proposed in order to increase the sensitivity and specificity of AKI diagnosis. Until the present, however, the benefit of those modifications in the clinical practice has not been clearly demonstrated.

---

[*] E-mail: jalopes93@hotmail.com

In this chapter we describe the AKI definition and staging according to the RIFLE and AKIN classifications, focusing on their main differences, advantages and limitations. We also review the more relevant studies validating such classifications in different settings of hospitalized patients.

Introduction

Although recent advances in the comprehension of the pathogenesis of acute kidney injury (AKI) and the modern therapies applied in this setting have been made, many issues related to AKI remain controversial and non-consensual. Over the last decades, more than 35 different definitions have been used to define AKI [1]. Many of those definitions were complex; however, the more commonly used were based on urine output (UO) and/or serum creatinine (SCr) criteria. An increase in basal SCr of at least 0.5 mg/dl, a decrease in Cr clearance of at least 50% or the need for renal replacement therapy (RRT) were the most frequent definitions used for AKI in clinical practice [2]. Whenever UO was used to define AKI, it has generally been considered a value lower than 400 to 500 ml per day as diagnostic criteria. Multiple definitions for AKI have obviously led to a great disparity in the reported incidence of AKI, making it difficult or even impossible to compare the various published studies focusing on AKI. For example, according to the definition employed, the previously described incidence of AKI in critically ill patients has varied between 1 and 25 percent and mortality has ranged from 15 to 60% [3, 4, 5, 6]. An adequate illustration of the influence of the definition used on the incidence of AKI and its associated mortality was demonstrated by Chertow and colleagues [7]. In this study, 9210 hospitalized patients with two or more determinations of SCr were evaluated. The incidence of AKI and in-hospital mortality were analyzed according to nine different definitions of AKI; the most sensitive defined AKI as an absolute increase in SCr equal or higher than 0.3 mg/dl, and the most specific defined AKI as an absolute increase in SCr equal or higher than 2.0 mg/dl. Taking into account the definition used, in this cohort of patients, the incidence of AKI varied between 1 e 40% and the relative risk for in-hospital death varied from 4.1 and 16.4. Therefore, it became crucial to establish a consensual and accurate definition of AKI that could desirably be used worldwide.

The Risk Injury Failure Loss of Kidney Function End-Stage Kidney Disease (RIFLE) Classification

In May 2002, the Acute Dialysis Quality Initiative (ADQI) group for the study of AKI, composed by nephrologists and intensivists, gathered during two days in a conference in Vicenza (Italy), with the purpose of defining AKI. From this conference, the consensual Risk Injury Failure Loss of kidney function End-stage kidney disease (RIFLE) classification for AKI definition emerged, and was later published in May 2004 on *Critical Care* [8].

The ADQI group considered that the ideal AKI definition would have to accomplish the following criteria: easy clinical applicability, sensitivity and specificity, consider baseline SCr variations, and also consider the "acute-on-chronic" phenomenon (which means the occurrence of an acute insult over a chronically injured renal function causing its deterioration). This definition should classify AKI according to its severity (mild versus severe) and its timing of occurrence (precocious versus late AKI). By fulfilling these criteria, this classification should allow the detection of patients whose kidney function was slightly affected (high sensitivity but low specificity) as well as patients with severe kidney function deterioration (high specificity with diminishing sensitivity). The RIFLE classification (Table 1) is based on SCr and UO determinations, and considers three severity classes of AKI (Risk, Injury, and Failure), according to the variations in SCr and/or UO, and two outcome classes (Loss of kidney function and End-stage kidney disease). The patient should be classified using the criteria (SCr and/or UO) which leads to the worst classification (maximum RIFLE), for instance, if a patient would be in Risk class according to UO but in Injury class according to SCr variation, then the worst criteria (SCr) should be used for classifying AKI in this patient. The temporal pattern of the SCr and/or UO variation is also relevant for defining AKI: the deterioration of renal function must be sudden (1 to 7 days) and sustained (persisting more than 24 hours). The Risk category is defined by an increase of at least 50% in baseline SCr or by a decrease in basal glomerular filtration rate (GFR) higher than 25%, or by a UO lower than 0.5 ml/kg/hour for more than 6 hours; Injury category is defined by an increase in baseline SCr of at least 100% or by a decrease in GFR higher than 50%, or by a UO lower than 0.5 ml/kg/hour for more than 12 hours; and Failure category is defined by an increase in baseline SCr of at least 200% or by a decrease in GFR higher than 75%, or by a UO lower than 0.3 ml/kg/hour for more than 24 hours or anuria for more than12 hours.

Table 1. Risk, Injury, Failure, Loss of kidney function, End-stage kidney disease (RIFLE) classification [8]. For the conversion of SCr expressed in conventional units into ST units, it should be multiplied by 88.4. To define AKI, the deterioration of renal function should be sudden (1 to 7 days) and sustained (persisting longer than 24 hours). Patients are classified based on SCr or UO or both, and the worst classification is considered. The variation in GFR is calculated according to SCr variation in reference to its baseline value. When baseline SCr is unknown and there in no history of chronic kidney disease, baseline SCr is calculated through the Modification of Diet in Renal Disease equation [9], assuming a GFR of 75 ml/min/1.73m^2

Class	GFR	UO
Risk	↑ SCr X 1.5 or ↓ GFR > 25%	< 0.5 ml/kg/h X 6h
Injury	↑ SCr X 2 or ↓ GFR > 50%	< 0.5 ml/kg/h X 12h
Failure	↑ SCr X 3 or ↓ GFR > 75% or if baseline SCr ≥ 4 mg/dl ↑ SCr > 0.5 mg/dl	< 0.3 ml/kg/h X 24h or anuria X 12h
Loss of kidney function	Complete loss of kidney function > 4 weeks	
End-stage kidney disease	Complete loss of kidney function > 3 months	

In those patients with baseline SCr higher than 4 mg/dl, Failure category is also defined by an increase in baseline SCr higher than 0.5 mg/dl. If this definition can easily be applied when baseline SCr is known, however, in a significant number of patients baseline SCr is unknown; in these cases, if there is no history of chronic kidney disease (CKD), baseline SCr should be calculated using the Modification of Diet in Renal Disease (MDRD) [9] equation, assuming a baseline GFR of 75 ml/min/1.73m^2.

Validation of the RIFLE Criteria

Following its publication, many studies have validated RIFLE classification in terms of determining the incidence of AKI and its prognostic stratification in several settings, such as hospitalized patients [10,11], Intensive Care Unit (ICU) patients [12, 13, 14, 15,16,17], patients undergoing cardiac surgery [18,19,20], patients with circulatory arrest induced by hypothermia to protect cerebrum during aortic arch surgery [21], patients submitted to abdominal aortic surgery [22], chirrotic patients [23], patients undergoing hepatic transplantation [24, 25], patients with sepsis [26, 27, 28], burn patients [29, 30,31,32], critically ill human immunodeficiency virus (HIV) infected patients [33], trauma patients [34] and patients receiving hematopoietic stem cell transplantation (HCT) [35]. Of interest, two studies have applied the RIFLE criteria to analyze the value of the serum cystatin C [36] and of the arterial resistivity index determined by Eco-Doppler [37] on the diagnosis of AKI in critically ill patients.

Hospitalized Patients

In a retrospective single-center study involving 20126 patients, 9.1% of them were in the Risk class for AKI, 5.2% were in the Injury class, and 3.7% were in the Failure class. There was an almost linear increase in in-hospital mortality from Normal to Failure class (Normal, 4.4%; Risk class, 15.1%; Injury class, 29.2%; and Failure class, 41.1%). Multivariate logistic regression analysis showed that all RIFLE criteria were significantly predictive factors for hospital mortality, with an almost linear increase in odds ratios (OR) from Risk to Failure classes (OR, Risk class 2.5, Injury class 5.4, and Failure class 10.1) [10]. Ali and colleagues performed a retrospective cohort study including 5321 hospitalized patients in the Grampian region of Scotland. A total of 474 patients (8.9%) were classified as having AKI (Risk class, 1.9%; Injury class, 4.4%; and Failure class, 2.6%). In-hospital mortality increased with severity of AKI (Risk class, 27%; Injury class, 30%; and Failure class, 41%; P=0.035) [11].

ICU Patients

Abosaif and colleagues retrospectively evaluated 183 critically ill patients and determined sensitivity and specificity of RIFLE classification in predicting mortality. Mortality in ICU (Risk class, 38.3%; Injury class, 50%; and Failure class, 74.5%) and mortality at 6 months after hospital discharge (Risk class, 43.3%; Injury class, 53.6%; and Failure class, 86%) were higher in patients in Failure class. These authors also found that

RIFLE classification improved the predictive ability of Acute Physiology and Chronic Health Evaluation score, version II (APACHE II) and Simplified Acute Physiology Score, version II (SAPS II) [12]. In a prospective study of 668 ICU patients, Ahlström and colleagues observed that maximum RIFLE within the first 3 days of hospitalization emerged as an independent predictor of in-hospital mortality and the discriminative power of RIFLE classification in mortality was moderate (AUROC = 0.653) [13]. In a multicenter and retrospective study, Hoste and colleagues analyzed 5383 patients admitted to 7 North American ICUs. AKI occurred in 67% of patients: 28% were in Risk class, 27% were in Injury class and 12% were in Failure class. During the ICU stay, 56% of patients in Risk class progressed to a more severe class (Injury or Failure classes). Patients with AKI had higher in-hospital mortality compared with patients who did not develop acute renal function deterioration, and it increased in accordance to AKI severity (no AKI, 5.5%; Risk class, 8.8%; Injury class, 11.4%; and Failure class, 26.3%). Multivariate analysis showed that all RIFLE classes were independently associated with in-hospital mortality [14]. Ostermann and Chang retrospectively studied 41972 patients admitted to 22 ICUs from United Kingdom and Germany, and observed that AKI defined by RIFLE classification occurred in 35.8% of patients (Risk class, 17.2%; Injury class, 11%; and Failure class, 7.6%). Similarly, patients with AKI were at increased risk for in-hospital mortality, and this risk increased as renal function deteriorated (no AKI, 8.4%; Risk class, 20.9%; Injury class, 45.6%; and Failure class, 56.8%). RIFLE classes were also independent predictors of in-hospital mortality [15]. Cruz and colleagues prospectively analyzed 2164 patients admitted to 19 ICUs of Northeast Italy. 10.8% of patients had AKI; 19% were in Risk class, 35% were in Injury class, and 46% in Failure class. Mortality was higher in Failure patients (Risk class, 20%; Injury class, 29.3%; and Failure class, 49.5%) and RIFLE classes were associated with mortality [16]. Bagshaw and colleagues used the Australian New Zealand Intensive Care Society Adult Patient Database and evaluated 120123 critically patients hospitalized at least 24 hours in 57 ICUs across Australia. At admission, 36.1% of patients had AKI (Risk class, 16.3%; Injury class, 13.6%; and Failure class, 6.3%). In-hospital mortality was 17.9% in Risk patients, 27.7% in Injury patients and 33.2% in Failure patients. RIFLE classes independently predicted mortality (OR: Risk class 1.58, Injury class 2.54 and Failure class 3.22) [17].

Patients Undergoing Cardiac Surgery

Heringlake and colleagues analyzed the incidence and stratification of AKI severity defined by RIFLE classification in 29623 patients undergoing cardiac surgery in 26 German centers. AKI in the post-operative period occurred in 16% of patients (Risk class, 9%; Injury class, 5%; and Failure class, 2%) [18]. Kuitunen and colleagues evaluated 813 patients submitted to cardiac surgery and found that 19.4% of patients had AKI in the post-operative period (Risk class, 10.9%; Injury class, 3.5%; and Failure class, 5%). Mortality at day 60 was higher in AKI patients, compared with patients who did not develop AKI, and it increased in accordance to AKI severity (no AKI, 0.9%; Risk, 8%; Injury, 21.4%; and Failure, 32.5%). RIFLE classification demonstrated a good prognostic accuracy (AUROC = 0.824) [19]. In a retrospective study of 46 critically ill patients (most had post-cardiotomy cardiogenic shock) treated by extracorporal membrane oxygenation, AKI occurred in 78.2% of patients (Risk class, 15.2%; Injury class, 39.1%; and Failure class, 23.9%). Injury and Failure classes were associated with increased in-hospital mortality (OR: Injury 10.40, and Failure infinitum) and RIFLE classification discriminated   mortality well in those patients (AUROC = 0.868). Cumulative survival rates at 6 months following hospital discharge differed significantly (P < 0.05) for non-AKI versus Injury and Failure classes, and Risk class versus Failure class [20].

Patients Undergoing Aortic Arch Surgery

A single-center and retrospective cohort study of 267 patients undergoing aortic arch surgery with deep hypothermic circulatory arrest was conducted by Arnaoutakis and colleagues. In the first week following surgery, 48% of patients developed AKI: 20% were in Risk class, 12% were in Injury class and 16% in Failure class. Mortality at day 30 was significantly higher in AKI patients and varied with AKI severity (no AKI, 3%; Risk class, 9%; Injury class, 12%; and Failure class, 38%) [21].

Patients Undergoing Abdominal Aortic Surgery

The RIFLE criteria were employed to define AKI in 69 patients submitted to elective abdominal aortic surgery. According to this classification, 22% of patients had AKI in the post-operative period and 33% of patients progressed to Failure class [22].

Chirrotic Patients

Jenq and colleagues [23] evaluated 134 critically ill chirrotic patients and observed that in-hospital mortality was higher in patients who developed AKI, compared to non-AKI patients, and it increased as renal function deteriorated (no AKI, 32.1%; Risk class, 68.8%; Injury class, 71.4%; and Failure class, 94.8%; P < 0.001). These authors also found that RIFLE classes were independent predictors of mortality (Risk class, OR 4.65; Injury class, OR 5.29; and Failure class, OR 38.82; P < 0.001). RIFLE classification, like the specific score for hepatic disease "Model for End-stage Liver Disease", as well as general severity scoring systems (APACHE II, APACHE III and Sequential Organ Failure Assessment), exhibited a good prognostic acuity (RIFLE, AUROC = 0.837, P < 0.001; Model for End-stage Liver Disease score, AUROC = 0.878, P < 0.001; APACHE II, AUROC = 0.810, P < 0.001; APACHE III, AUROC = 0.885, P < 0.001; and Sequential Organ Failure Assessment, AUROC = 0.917, P < 0.001).

Patients Submitted to Hepatic Transplantation

In a retrospective study performed by Guitard and colleagues that evaluated 94 patients receiving a hepatic graft, AKI occurred in 63.8% of patients (41.5% were in Injury class and 22.3% were in Failure class). AKI was associated with increased mortality at 1-year of follow-up [24]. O'Riordan and colleagues retrospectively studied 359 patients who were submitted to hepatic transplantation and found that AKI occurred in 35.9% of cases: 10.9% of patients were in Injury class and 25% were in Failure class. Failure patients had lower survival at 30 days and 1-year after transplantation (P < 0.001) [25].

Septic Patients

In a single-center Portuguese study, Lopes and colleagues retrospectively analyzed 182 critically ill patients with sepsis. The incidence of AKI was 37.4% (6% of patients were in Risk class, 11.6% were in Injury class and 19.8% in Failure class). Mortality on day 60 was significantly higher in AKI patients, as compared with patients with no AKI, and it increased in accordance to AKI severity (normal renal function, 9.6%; Risk class, 27.3%; Injury class, 28.6%; and Failure class, 55%; P < 0.0001). On multivariate analysis, Failure class (OR 3.59, 95% CI 1.44 - 8.94, P = 0.006) emerged as independent predictor of mortality. The RIFLE predicted well mortality in septic patients (AUROC = 0.750 ± 0.047; P < 0.0001) [26]. In a retrospective study of prospectively collected data from the Australian New Zealand Intensive Care Society Adult Patient Database involving 33375 patients with sepsis from 57 ICUs across Australia, 42.1% had concomitant AKI. Thirty-eight and five percent of patients belonged to the Risk class, 38.8% to the Injury class and 22.7% to the Failure class. [27]. In-hospital mortality was higher in AKI patients, compared with patients with no AKI, and it increased with AKI severity (normal renal function, 12.6%; Risk class, 23.4%; Injury class, 32.2%; and Failure class, 35.8%). In a single-center study evaluating 121 critically ill patients with sepsis, the incidence of AKI was 56.1% (Risk class, 26.4%; Injury class, 15.7%; and Failure class, 14%). In-hospital mortality was 34% for non-AKI patients, 40.6% for Risk patients, 73.7% for Injury patients, and 76.5% for Failure patients (P < 0.001). In all patients, RIFLE severity correlated with mortality. Odds ratios for RIFLE criteria were 1.33 (P = 0.537) for Risk class versus non-AKI, 5.444 (P = 0.004) for Injury class versus non-AKI, and 6.319 (P = 0.004) for Failure class versus non-AKI. In all patients, RIFLE severity correlated with mortality. The AUROC for RIFLE was 0.678 (P = 0.001). Cumulative survival rates at 6 months of follow-up differed significantly (P < 0.05) for non-AKI versus Injury and Failure classes, and for Risk class versus Failure class [28].

Burn Patients

In a retrospective study, Coca and colleagues found that 26.6% of 304 patients with total burned surface area equal or higher than 10% developed AKI. In-hospital mortality was higher in Failure patients, although in-hospital mortality was similar between Risk, Injury and non-AKI patients [29]. In a singler-center study from Portugal, 126 patients with severe burns were retrospectively evaluated. During hospitalization, 35.7% of patients developed AKI: 14.3% were in Risk class, 8.7% were in Injury class and 12.7% in Failure class. In-hospital mortality was higher in AKI patients, compared with patients with no AKI, and it increased according to AKI severity (normal renal function, 6%; Risk class, 11.1%; Injury class, 63.6%; and Failure class, 75%; P < 0.0001). After adjusting for other covariates, Risk and Injury classes (Risk class OR 5.6, 95% CI 1.2 - 26.8, P < 0.0001; Injury class OR 6.2, 95% CI 1.1 - 47.8, P = 0.008) were both independent predictors of mortality. The RIFLE classification had a good prognostic accuracy (AUROC = 0.843 ± 0.051; P < 0.0001) [30]. In a single-center and prospective study, Steinvall and colleagues determined the incidence and outcome of AKI after major burns (total burned surface area of 20% or more). Of 127 patients, 31 (24%) developed AKI (12% Risk class, 8% Injury class, and 5% Failure class). Mortality was 14% and increased with increasing RIFLE class (7% normal, 13% Risk class, 40% Injury class, and 83% Failure class) [31]. In a retrospective and single-center cohort study of 60 patients with a burn injury of 20% or more of total body surface area, 53.3% of them developed AKI: Risk class in 28.1%, Injury class in 18.8% and Failure class in 53.1%. Patients with AKI had a mortality rate of 34.4%. None of the patients who did not develop AKI during ICU stay died. Thirteen patients progressed to higher class of AKI. Patients who progressed to higher RIFLE class had higher mortality rate (46%) compared to those who remained at the same class (Risk or Injury classes) (7.7%). Logistic regression analysis indicated that Failure class of AKI (P = 0.033) was an independent risk factor for mortality [32].

Critically Ill Human Immunodeficiency Virus Infected Patients

Lopes and colleagues retrospectively evaluated 97 critically ill HIV infected patients and observed that, according to the RIFLE, 46 patients (47.4%) developed AKI: 12.4% were in Risk class, 9.2% were in Injury class and 25.8% in Failure class. Mortality on day 60 was significantly higher in AKI patients, compared with patients with no AKI, and it increased in accordance to AKI severity (normal renal function, 23.5%; Risk class, 50%; Injury class, 66.6%; and Failure class, 72%; P < 0.0001). Multivariate analysis showed that Injury and Failure classes (Injury class OR 5.12, 95% CI 1.07 - 24.28, P = 0.04; and Failure class OR 4.6, 95% CI 1.57 - 13.5, P = 0.005) were both independent predictors of mortality. The RIFLE exhibited a good capacity in predicting mortality (AUROC = 0.732 ± 0.053; P < 0.0001) [33].

Trauma Patients

In a retrospective interrogation of prospectively collected data from the Australian New Zealand Intensive Care Society Adult Patient Database, Bagshaw and colleagues evaluated the incidence and outcomes associated with early AKI (evident within 24 hours of admission) in critically ill trauma patients. A total of 9449 patients were admitted for more than 24 hours to 57 ICUs across Australia. The crude incidence of AKI was 18.1%, and it was associated with a higher crude mortality (16.7% vs. 7.8%, OR 2.36, 95% CI, 2.0-2.7, P < 0.001). Each RIFLE class of AKI was independently associated with hospital mortality in multi-variable analysis (Risk class: OR 1.69; Injury class OR 1.88; and Failure class 2.29) [34].

Patients Receiving Hematopoietic Stem Cell Transplantation

In a retrospective and single-center study involving 82 patients who underwent a reduced intensity conditioning (RIC) HCT, Lopes and colleagues found that 53.6% developed AKI within the first 100 days after HCT: 25% were in Risk class, 45.5% were in Injury class and

29.5% in Failure class. In all, 64 patients survived after 100 days of post-transplant and were available for long-term survival analysis. At follow-up, 43.7% of patients died. A 5-year overall survival of AKI patients was 41.6% as compared with 67.1% for those who did not develop AKI (P = 0.028), and decreased according to AKI severity (Risk class, 55.6%; Injury plus Failure classes, 33.3%; P = 0.045). After controlling for other covariates, AKI predicted 5-year overall mortality (AKI: adjusted hazard ratio, 2.36, 95% CI: 1.03-5.37; P = 0.041). Moreover, moderate and severe AKI (Injury plus Failure classes) was also associated with an increased 5-year overall mortality (Injury plus Failure classes: adjusted hazard ratio, 1.64, 95% CI: 1.06-2.54; P = 0.024) [35].

Strenghts and Weaknesses of the RIFLE Classification

Strenghts of the RIFLE Classification

These studies have shown that AKI is frequent in hospitalized patients, particularly in ICU patients, and it is associated with increased morbidity and mortality. In addition, it has been demonstrated that mortality increased in accordance to AKI severity, and RIFLE had a good prognostic accuracy. It has simultaneously been shown that the RIFLE allows monitoring the progression of AKI severity within hospitalization in the ICU [14, 38]. Originally, the RIFLE criteria have been established to uniformize the definition and stratification of AKI severity. Several studies, however, have determined the ability of the RIFLE in predicting mortality using the AUROC curve, and some of them have inclusively compared it with other general or specific scoring systems [12, 13, 19, 20, 26, 30, 33].

Taking into account that RIFLE relies only in renal function, it would be expected that RIFLE prognostic capacity was inferior to that of other scores (i.e. APACHE, SAPS). The RIFLE has shown to be an important tool to predict patient outcome and, furthermore, it seemed to increase the prognostic ability of other general scores usually employed in the ICUs (i.e. APACHE, SAPS).

Weaknesses of the RIFLE Classification

Despite its clinical utility, the RIFLE classication has some important limitations. First, baseline SCr is necessary to define and classify AKI. However, this baseline value is frequently unknown in clinical practice. In order to obviate this concern, the ADQI workgroup [8] have proposed to estimate baseline SCr using the MDRD equation [9], assuming a baseline GFR of 75 ml/min/1.73m^2. In CKD patients, baseline SCr determined assuming a GFR of 75 ml/min/1.73m^2 has a low correlation with the real value of SCr and it results in an overestimation of AKI incidence [39]. Second, the MDRD formula has been validated in CKD patients with stable renal function, not in AKI patients. Third, in several of the studies previously mentioned, only SCr was used to define and stage AKI [15, 18, 24, 25, 38]. In CKD patients, compared with patients with previously normal renal function, the percentual increase in SCr used to define AKI generally occurs later and, thus, defining AKI by employing exclusively SCr criteria could diminish sensitivity of AKI diagnosis in CKD patients [40]. Moreover, determining renal function using SCr has other several limitations, as follow:

a) the endogenous production and serum release of Cr is variable, and it is influenced by multiple factors, namely age, gender, diet, and muscle mass;
b) 10 to 40% of Cr elimination is performed by tubular secretion [41] and this mechanism is amplified as GFR diminishes, thus, overestimating renal function in AKI patients;
c) many medications inhibit tubular secretion of Cr (i.e. thrimetroprim, cimetidine), causing a temporary increase in SCr;
d) various factors can interfere with SCr determination (i.e. acetoacetate accumulated in diabetic cetoacidosis can interfer with the alcaline picrate method), originating a false elevation in SCr [42];
e) Cr is a marker of renal function, and not of renal lesion.

Fifth, decrease in UO is sensitive and frequent in AKI, however, it also has some important limitations in defining and staging AKI [43]:

a) sensitivity and specificity of UO can be significantly changed by diuretics use, and this issue is not specifically considered in RIFLE classification;
b) UO can only be determined in patients with a bladder catheter in place, which, despite being common in ICU patients, is not frequent in other hospitalized patients;
c) It is possible that predictive ability of UO could be inferior to that of SCr, which can explain the difference in terms of mortality between the same classes defined by each one of those criteria, observed in the studies that utilized both criteria to define and classify AKI [14, 16, 44]. The capacity of the RIFLE (using both criteria) to predict mortality can be more stable than the ability of this classification employing only SCr [16], which corroborates the clinical utility of using both criteria as proposed by the ADQI workgroup simultaneously [8].

Sixth, the etiology of AKI and the requirement for RRT is not considered in RIFLE classification. In two studies that evaluated ICU patients with AKI requiring hemodialysis, RIFLE classification has shown less acuity in predicting mortality [45, 46]. Bell and colleagues evaluated 207 critically ill patients with AKI undergoing continuous RRT. 60-day mortality was 23.5% in patients in Risk class, 22% in patients in Injury class and 57.9% in patients in Failure class [45]. Maccariello and colleagues prospectively evaluated 179 ICU patients receiving continuous RRT: 25% of patients were in Risk class, 27% were in Injury class and 48% in Failure class. These authors did not find any statistically significant difference in mortality between RIFLE classes (Risk class, 72%; Injury class, 79%; and Failure class, 76%). On multivariate analysis, RIFLE classes were not associated with mortality [46]. One possible explanation for this phenomenon is that in both studies, clinical severity of patients was so high that it could not allow RIFLE to discriminate mortality according to AKI severity (i.e. between the three classes). Last, RIFLE classification does not provide any information regarding the origin of the renal lesion (i.e. cellular or subcelular levels), as opposed to several biomarkers of AKI recently identified and studied. Furthermore, the limitations of the conventional renal function markers (Cr and UO) can be overwhelmed with the utilization of those new biomarkers. In fact, various urinary and serum markers of AKI have been identified and described [47], such as neutrophil gelatinase-associated lipocalin (NGAL), interleucine-18 (IL-18) and the kidney injury molecule-1 (KIM-1). These biomarkers start to elevate soon in AKI (1 to 3 days before the increase in SCr), and do exhibit a great sensitivity and specificity in AKI diagnosis, a good correlation with RRT requirement, as well as with mortality, in several settings, namely in the post-operative period of cardiac surgery [48, 49, 50, 51], in ICU patients [52, 53] and in the contrast-induced nephropathy in children undergoing cardiac catheterism [54]. In renal transplantation, it has been shown that these biomarkers also have a good correlation with the cold ischemic time, the maximum value of SCr in the post-transplantation period and the requirement for RRT, and also predicts acute tubular necrosis and long-term function of renal graft well[55, 56, 57, 58]. It must also be emphasized that RIFLE criteria have only been evaluated in a minority (< 2 %) of patients included in prospective studies. This major concern certainly did limit the analysis of other clinical or laboratory variables with prognostic impact in the epidemiology of AKI.

The Acute Kidney Injury Network (AKIN) classification

In September 2005, in a meeting in Amsterdam, a new classification of AKI has been proposed by the Acute Kidney Injury Network (AKIN) working group composed of nephrologists, critical care physicians and other physicians specialized in AKI. The AKIN classification (Table 2) has been published in Marrch 2007 on *Critical Care* [59], and it is a version of RIFLE classification with some modifications: the diagnosis of AKI is only considered after achieving an adequate status of hydration and after excluding urinary obstruction; the AKIN classification only relies in SCr and not in GFR changes; baseline SCr is not necessary in AKIN classification, and it requires at least two values of SCr obtained within a period of 48 hours; AKI is defined by the sudden decrease (in 48 hours) of renal function, defined by an increase in absolute SCr of at least 0.3 mg/dl or by a percentual increase in SCr equal or higher than 50% (1.5x baseline value), or by a decrease in UO (documented oliguria lower than 0.5 ml/kg/hour for more than 6 hours); stage 1 corresponds to Risk class, but it also considers an absolute increase in SCr equal or higher than 0.3 mg/dl; stages 2 and 3 correspond to Injury and Failure classes, respectively; stage 3 also considers patients requiring RRT independently of the stage (defined by SCr and/or UO) they are in at the moment they initiate RRT; the two outcome classes (Loss of kidney function and End-stage kidney disease) were removed from the classification. These modifications were based in the cumulative evidence that even small increases in SCr are associated with a poor outcome, and in the extreme variability of resources and of the indications to start RRT exhibited in different countries and hospitals. Levy and colleagues demonstrated that an increase in baseline SCr equal or higher than 25% within two days following administration of contrast media was associated with a risk of death of 5.5 [60]. Lassnigg and colleagues showed that even a mild increase (0 a 0.5 mg/dl) in baseline SCr in the post-operative period of cardiac surgery was associated with a 3-fold risk of death within 30 days [61]. In 2005,

Chertow and colleagues demonstrated that an increase in SCr equal or higher than 0.3 mg/dl within the hospitalization increased the risk of death by 4.1-fold [7]. After its publication, two studies have shown that an absolute increase in SCr equal or higher than 0.3 mg/dl within 48 hours increased length   of hospitalization and in-hospital mortality both in hospitalized patients and in the ICU setting [62, 63]. Barrantes and colleagues evaluated 735 patients with AKI defined as an increase in the SCr level of 0.3 mg/dl or more within 48 hours and 5089 controls admitted to a North American community teaching hospital. Overall, patients with AKI had higher in-hospital mortality (14.8% versus 1.5%; P < 0.001), longer lengths of stay (median 7.9 versus 3.7 days; P < 0.001), and higher rates of transfer to critical care areas (28.6% versus 4.3%; P < 0.001); survivors were more likely to be discharged to an extended care facility (43.1% versus 20.3%; P < 0.001). Conditional multivariate logistic regression analyses of the 282 pairs of cases and controls showed that patients with AKI were 8 times more likely to die in a hospital (OR 7.9; 95% CI 2.9-15.3) and were 5 times more likely to have prolonged (> or = 7 days) hospital stays (OR 5.2, 95% CI 3.5-7.9) and require intensive care (OR 4.7, 95% CI 2.7-8.1), after adjustment for age, comorbidities, and other potential confounders [62].

In a retrospective cohort study of 471 ICU patients, 45.2% had an increment equal to or higher than 0.3 mg/dl in SCr within 48 hours and/or UO equal or lower than 0.5 ml/kg/hours for more than 6 hours. The mortality rate of patients who met criteria for AKI was significantly higher than that of patients who did not have AKI (45.8 versus 16.4%, P < 0.01). In multivariate logistic regression analyses, AKI was an independent predictor of mortality (OR 3.7, 95% CI 2.2-6.1). Median hospital stay was twice as long in patients with AKI (14 versus 7 days, P < 0.01) [63]. The AKIN classification could theoretically improve the RIFLE criteria sensitivity and specificity, although the advantages of the RIFLE modifications have not been proven yet [44, 64, 65]. Lopes and colleagues demonstrated in a single-cohort study of 662 ICU patients that AKIN classification compared to RIFLE classification did not show a better prognostic acuity in terms of in-hospital mortality, although it allowed the identification of 6.6% more patients as having AKI (P = 0.018) [44].

In a multicentric study involving 120123 patients admitted to 57 ICUs across Australia there were no differences in the incidence of AKI within the first 24 hours of hospitalization and in hospital mortality, when patients were classified according to both classifications [64]. Moreover, in a multicentric study evaluating 16784 critically ill patients using the SAPS 3 database, the RIFLE criteria demonstrated higher diagnostic sensitivity and predictive value of mortality than AKIN classification. [65]. These results suggest that the modifications proposed to RIFLE, the most widely used classification for AKI by the nephrological and intensive care community, do not improve the ability of this classification in predicting mortality of critically ill patients [66].

Strengths and Weaknesses of the AKIN Classification

Taking into account that AKIN classification is a modified version of the RIFLE classification, their strenghs and limitations are very similar to those aforementioned for the

RIFLE. The AKIN classification has, however, some additional benefits and limitations related to the modifications themselves introduced to RIFLE classification.

Table 2. Classification / staging system of AKI [61] based on RIFLE classification [8]. AKI is defined by the sudden decrease (in 48 houres) of renal function, defined by an increase in absolute SCr of at least 0.3 mg/dl or by a percentual increase in SCr equal or higher than 50% (1.5x baseline value), or by a decrease in UO (documented oliguria lower than 0.5 ml/kg/h for more than 6 hours); [a]stage 3 also includes patients requiring renal replacement therapy (RRT) independently of the stage (defined by SCr and/or UO) they are in at the moment they initiate RRT

Stage	SCr	UO
1	↑ SCr ≥ 0.3 mg/dl or ↑ SCr ≥ 150 a 200% (1.5 a 2 X)	< 0.5 ml/kg/h (> 6h)
2	↑ SCr > 200 a 300% (> 2 a 3 X)	< 0.5 ml/kg/h (> 12h)
3[a]	↑ SCr > 300% (> 3 X) or if baseline SCr ≥ 4.0 mg/dl ↑ SCrS ≥ 0.5 mg/dl	< 0.3 ml/kg/h (24h) or anuria (12h)

Strengths of the AKIN Classification

First, AKI definition is only considered after an adequate status of hydration is achieved. Furthermore, the AKIN classification, unlikely RIFLE, adds important etiological information. Second, AKIN classification is based in SCr and not in GFR changes. Third, AKIN classification does not need baseline SCr to define AKI, although it requires at least two SCr determinations within 48 hours.

Weaknesses of the AKIN Classification

First, the AKIN classification does not allow the identification of AKI when SCr elevation occurs in a frametime higher than 48 hours. Second, stage 3 of AKIN classification includes three diagnostic criteria (Cr, UO, and RRT requirement), and the extreme variability in the beginning and cessation of RRT as well as in RRT modality used and in dose of dialysis among different physicians, hospitals and countries could significantly limit the prognostic acuity of this classification, particularly of stage 3.

Which Classification Should We Use in Clinical Practice?

The extensive number of publications focusing on RIFLE and AKIN classifications are demonstrative. They are widely accepted by the medical community and, therefore, we strongly recommend the utilization of either one or the other to define AKI and classify its severity. It persists, however, some heterogeneity in the utilization of the criteria defining and classifying AKI, such as the use or not of UO and baseline SCr, and of estimated GFR instead of the variation in SCr.

Taking into account the aforementioned limitations, it is of remarkable importance to assume there is still not a perfect definition of AKI. In the future, it will be reasonable to make the fusion of both classifications in order to establish only one classification of AKI that would be uniformly utilized. Furthermore, it is proposed to employ an absolute increase in SCr equal or higher than 0.3 mg/dl in a timeframe higher than 48 hours. Moreover, the integration of the new biomarkers of AKI into the clinical classification could increase sensitivity and specificity of AKI diagnosis, overwhelming some of the limitations of the traditional markers of kidney function, such as Cr and UO [67].

References

[1]   Kellum JA, Levin N, Bouman C, Lameire N. Developing a consensus classification system for acute renal failure. *Curr. Opin. Crit. Care.* 2002; 8: 509-514.

[2]   Thadhani R, Pascual M, Bonventre JV. Acute renal failure. *N. Engl. J. Med.* 1996; 334: 1448-1460.

[3]   Schaefer JH, Jochimsen F, Keller F, Wegscheider K, Distler A. Outcome prediction of acute renal failure in medical intensive care. *Intensive Care Med.* 1991; 17: 19-24.

[4]   Brivet FG, Kleinknecht DJ, Loriat P, Landais PJ. Acute renal failure in intensive care units – causes, outcome, and prognostic factors of hospital mortality: a prospective, multi-center study. *Crit. Care Med.* 1996; 24: 192-198.

[5]   Liano F, Pascual J; Madrid Acute Renal Failure Study Cluster. Epidemiology of acute renal failure: a prospective, multi-center, community-based study. *Kidney Int.* 1996; 50: 811-818

[6]   Silvester W, Bellomo R, Cole L. Epidemiology, management, and outcome of severe acute renal failure of critical illness in Australia. *Crit. Care Med.* 2001; 29: 1910-1915.

[7]   Chertow GM, Burdick E, Honour M, Bonventre JV, Bates DW. Acute kidney injury, mortality, length of stay, and costs in hospitalized patients. *J. Am. Soc. Nephrol.* 2005; 16: 3365-3370.

[8]   Bellomo R, Ronco C, Kellum JA, Mehta RL, Palevsky P and the ADQI workgroup. Acute renal failure – definition, outcome measures, animal models, fluid therapy and information technology needs: the Second International Consensus Conference of the Acute Dialysis Quality Initiative (ADQI) Group. *Crit. Care,* 2004; 8: R204.

[9]   Manjunath G, Sarnak MJ, Levey AS. Prediction equations to estimate glomerular filtration rate: an update. *Curr. Opin. Nephrol. Hypertens,* 2001; 10: 785-792.

[10] Uchino S, Bellomo R, Goldsmith D, Bates S, Ronco C. An assessment of the RIFLE criteria for acute renal failure in hospitalized patients. *Crit. Care Med.* 2006; 34: 1913-1917.

[11] Ali T, Khan I, Simpson W, Prescott G, Townend J, Smith W, Macleod A. Incidence and outcomes in acute kidney injury: a comprehensive population-based study. *J. Am. Soc. Nephrol.* 2007; 18: 1292-1298.

[12] Abosaif NY, Tolba YA, Heap M, Russell J, El Nahas AM. The outcome of acute renal failure in the intensive care unit according to RIFLE: model application, sensitivity, and predictability. *Am. J. Kidney Dis.* 2005; 46: 1038-1048.

[13] Ahlström A, Kuitunen A, Peltonen S, Hynninen M, Tallgren M, Aaltonen J, Pettilä V. Comparison of 2 acute renal failure severity scores to general scoring systems in the critically ill. *Am. J. Kidney Dis.* 2006; 48: 262-268.

[14] Hoste EA, Clermont G, Kersten A, Venkataraman R, Angus DC, De Bacquer D, Kellum JA. RIFLE criteria for acute kidney injury are associated with hospital mortality in critically ill patients: a cohort analysis. *Crit. Care,* 2006; 10: R73.

[15] Ostermann M, Chang RW. Acute kidney injury in the intensive care unit according to RIFLE. *Crit. Care Med.* 2007; 35: 1837-1843.

[16] Cruz DN, Bolgan I, Perazella MA, Bonello M, de Cal M, Corradi V, Polanco N, Ocampo C, Nalesso F, Piccinni P, Ronco C; for the North East Italian Prospective Hospital Renal Outcome Survey on Acute Kidney Injury (NEiPHROS-AKI) Investigators. North East Italian Prospective Hospital Renal Outcome Survey on Acute Kidney Injury (NEiPHROS-AKI): targeting the problem with the RIFLE criteria. *Clin. J. Am. Soc. Nephrol.* 2007; 2: 418-425.

[17] Bagshaw SM, George C, Dinu I, Bellomo R. A multi-center evaluation of the RIFLE criteria for early acute kidney injury in critically ill patients. *Nephrol. Dial. Transplant.* 2008; 23: 1203-1210.

[18] Heringlake M, Knappe M, Vargas Hein O, Lufft H, Kindgen-Milles D, Böttiger BW, Weigand MR, Klaus S, Schirmer U. Renal dysfunction according to the ADQI-RIFLE system and clinical practice patterns after cardiac surgery in Germany. *Minerva Anestesiol.* 2006; 72: 645-654.

[19] Kuitunen A, Vento A, Suojaranta-Ylinen R, Pettilä V. Acute renal failure after cardiac surgery: evaluation of the RIFLE classification. *Ann. Thorac. Surg.* 2006; 81: 542-546.

[20] Lin CY, Chen YC, Tsai FC, Tian YC, Jenq CC, Fang JT, Yang CW. RIFLE classification is predictive of short-term prognosis in critically ill patients with acute renal failure supported by extracorporeal membrane oxygenation. *Nephrol. Dial. Transplant.* 2006; 21: 2867-2873.

[21] Arnaoutakis GJ, Bihorac A, Martin TD, Hess PJ Jr, Klodell CT, Ejaz AA, Garvan C, Tribble CG, Beaver TM. RIFLE criteria for acute kidney injury in aortic arch surgery. *J. Thorac. Cardiovasc. Surg.* 2007; 134: 1554-1560.

[22] Tallgren M, Niemi T, Pöyhiä R, Raininko E, Railo M, Salmenperä M, Lepäntalo M, Hynninen M. Acute renal injury and dysfunction following elective abdominal aortic surgery. *Eur. J. Vasc. Endovasc. Surg.* 2007; 33: 550-555.

[23] Jenq CC, Tsai MH, Tian YC, Lin CY, Yang C, Liu NJ, Lien JM, Chen YC, Fang JT, Chen PC, Yang CW. RIFLE classification can predict short-term prognosis in critically ill cirrhotic patients. *Intensive Care Med.* 2007; 33: 1921-1930.

[24] Guitard J, Cointault O, Kamar N, Muscari F, Lavayssière L, Suc B, Ribes D, Esposito L, Barange K, Durand D, Rostaing L. Acute renal failure following liver transplantation with induction therapy. *Clin. Nephrol.* 2006; 65: 103-112.

[25] O'Riordan A, Wong V, McQuillan R, McCormick PA, Hegarty JE, Watson AJ. Acute renal disease, as defined by the RIFLE criteria, post-liver transplantation. *Am. J. Transplant,* 2007; 7: 168-176.

[26] Lopes JA, Jorge S, Resina C, Santos C, Pereira A, Neves J, Antunes F, Prata MM. Prognostic utility of RIFLE for acute renal failure in patients with sepsis. *Crit. Care,* 2007; 11: 408.

[27] Bagshaw SM, George C, Bellomo R; ANZICS Database Management Committee. Early acute kidney injury and sepsis: a multi-center evaluation. *Crit Care* 2008; 12: R47

[28] Chen YC, Jenq CC, Tian YC, Chang MY, Lin CY, Chang CC, Lin HC, Fang JT, Yang CW, Lin SM. Rifle classification for predicting in-hospital mortality in critically ill sepsis patients. *Shock,* 2009; 31: 139-145.

[29] Coca SG, Bauling P, Schifftner T, Howard CS, Teitelbaum I, Parikh CR. Contribution of acute kidney injury toward morbidity and mortality in burns: a contemporary analysis. *Am. J. Kidney Dis.* 2007; 49: 517-523.

[30] Lopes JA, Jorge S, Neves FC, Caneira M, Gomes da Costa A, Cordeiro Ferreira A, Prata MM. An assessment of the RIFLE criteria for acute renal failure in severely burned patients. *Nephrol. Dial. Transplant.* 2007; 22: 285.

[31] Steinvall I, Bak Z, Sjoberg F. Acute kidney injury is common, parallels organ dysfunction or failure, and carries appreciable mortality in patients with major burns: a prospective exploratory cohort study. *Crit. Care,* 2008; 12: R124.

[32] Palmieri T, Lavrentieva A, Greenhalgh DG. Acute kidney injury in critically ill burn patients. Risk factors, progression and impact on mortality. *Burns,* 2010; 36: 205-211.

[33] Lopes JA, Fernandes J, Jorge S, Neves J, Antunes F, Prata MM. An assessment of the RIFLE criteria for acute renal failure in critically ill HIV-infected patients. *Crit. Care,* 2007; 11: 401.

[34] Bagshaw SM, George C, Gibney RT, Bellomo R. A multi-center evaluation of early acute kidney injury in critically ill trauma patients. *Ren. Fail.* 2008; 30: 581-589.

[35] Lopes JA, Gonçalves S, Jorge S, Raimundo M, Resende L, Lourenço F, Lacerda JF, Martins C, Carmo JA, Forjaz Lacerda JM, Prata MM. Contemporary analysis of the influence of the acute kidney injury after reduced intensity conditioning haematopoietic cell transplantation on long-term survival. *Bone Marrow Transplant.* 2008; 42: 619-626.

[36] Herget-Rosenthal S, Feldkamp T, Volbracht L, Kribben A. Measurement of urinary cystatin C by particle-enhanced nephelometric immunoassay: precision, interferences, stability and reference range. *Ann. Clin. Biochem.* 2004; 41: 111-118.

[37] Lerolle N, Guérot E, Faisy C, Bornstain C, Diehl JL, Fagon JY. Renal failure in septic shock: predictive value of Doppler-based renal arterial resistive index. *Intensive Care Med.* 2006; 32: 1553-1559.

[38] Lopes JA, Jorge S, Resina C, Santos C, Pereira A, Neves J, Antunes F, Prata MM. Acute kidney injury in patients with sepsis: a contemporary analysis. *Int. J. Infect. Dis.* 2009; 13: 176-181.

[39] Bagshaw SM, Uchino S, Cruz D, Bellomo R, Morimatsu H, Morgera S, Schetz M, Tan I, Bouman C, Macedo E, Gibney N, Tolwani A, Oudemans-van Straaten HM, Ronco C, Kellum JA; Beginning and Ending Supportive Therapy for the Kidney (BEST Kidney) Investigators. A comparison of observed versus estimated baseline creatinine for determination of RIFLE class in patients with acute kidney injury. *Nephrol. Dial. Transplant.* 2009; 24: 2739-2744.

[40] Waikar SS, Bonventre JV. Creatinine kinetics and the definition of acute kidney injury. *J. Am. Soc. Nephrol.* 2009; 20: 672-679.

[41] Shemesh O, Golbetz H, Kriss JP, Myers BD. Limitations of creatinine as a filtration marker in glomerulopathic patients. *Kidney Int.* 1985; 28: 830-838.

[42] Molitch ME, Rodman E, Hirsch CA, Dubinsky E. Spurious serum creatinine elevations in ketoacidosis. *Ann. Intern. Med.* 1980; 93: 280-281.

[43] Hoste EA, Kellum JA. Acute kidney injury: epidemiology and diagnostic criteria. *Curr. Opin. Crit. Care,* 2006; 12: 531-537.

[44] Lopes JA, Fernandes P, Jorge S, Gonçalves S, Alvarez A, Costa e Silva Z, França C, Martins Prata M. Acute kidney injury in intensive care unit patients: a comparison between the RIFLE and the Acute Kidney Injury Network classifications. *Crit. Care,* 2008; 12: R110.

[45] Bell M, Liljestam E, Granath F, Fryckstedt J, Ekbom A, Martling CR. Optimal follow-up time after continuous renal replacement therapy in actual renal failure patients stratified with the RIFLE criteria. *Nephrol. Dial. Transplant.* 2005; 20: 354-360.

[46] Maccariello E, Soares M, Valente C, Nogueira L, Valença RV, Machado JE, Rocha E. RIFLE classification in patients with acute kidney injury in need of renal replacement therapy. *Intensive Care Med.* 2007; 33: 597-605.

[47] Venkataraman R, Kellum JA. Defining acute renal failure: the RIFLE criteria. *J. Intensive Care Med.* 2007; 22: 187-193.

[48] Mishra J, Dent C, Tarabishi R, Mitsnefes MM, Ma Q, Kelly C, Ruff SM, Zahedi K, Shao M, Bean J, Mori K, Barasch J, Devarajan P. Neutrophil gelatinase associated lipocalin (NGAL) as a biomarker for acute renal injury after cardiac surgery. *Lancet* 2005; 365: 1231-1238.

[49] Parikh CR, Mishra J, Thiessen-Philbrook H, Dursun B, Ma Q, Kelly C, Dent C, Devarajan P, Edelstein CL. Urinary IL-18 is an early predictive biomarker of acute kidney injury after cardiac surgery. *Kidney Int.* 2006; 70: 199-203.

[50] Wagener G, Jan M, Kim M, Mori K, Barasch JM, Sladen RN, Lee HT. Association between increases in urinary neutrophil gelatinase-associated lipocalin and acute renal dysfunction after adult cardiac surgery. *Anesthesiology* 2006; 105: 485-491.

[51] Han WK, Waikar SS, Johnson A, Betensky RA, Dent CL, Devarajan P, Bonventre JV. Urinary biomarkers in the early diagnosis of acute kidney injury. *Kidney Int.* 2008; 73: 863-869.

[52] Parikh CR, Abraham E, Ancukiewicz M, Edelstein CL. Urine IL-18 is an early diagnostic marker for acute kidney injury and predicts mortality in the intensive care unit. *J. Am. Soc. Nephrol.* 2005; 16: 3046-3052.

[53] Liangos O, Perianayagam MC, Vaidya VS, Han WK, Wald R, Tighiouart H, MacKinnon RW, Li L, Balakrishnan VS, Pereira BJ, Bonventre JV, Jaber BL. Urinary *N*-acetyl-beta-D glucosaminidase activity and kidney injury molecule-1 level are

associated with adverse outcomes in acute renal failure. *J. Am. Soc. Nephrol.* 2007; 18: 904-912.

[54] Hirsch R, Dent C, Pfriem H, Allen J, Beekman RH 3rd, Ma Q, Dastrala S, Bennett M, Mitsnefes M, Devarajan P. NGAL is an early predictive biomarker of contrast induced nephropathy in children. *Pediatr. Nephrol.* 2007; 22: 2089-2095.

[55] Mishra J, Ma Q, Kelly C, Mitsnefes M, Mori K, Barasch J, Devarajan P. Kidney NGAL is a novel early marker of acute injury following transplantation. *Pediatr. Nephrol.* 2006; 21: 856-863.

[56] Parikh CR, Jani A, Melnikov VY, Faubel S, Edelstein C. Urinary interleukin-18 is a marker of human acute tubular necrosis. *Am. J. Kidney Dis.* 2004; 43: 405-414.

[57] Parikh CR, Jani A, Mishra J, Ma Q, Kelly C, Barasch J, Edelstein CL, Devarajan P. Urine NGAL and IL-18 are predictive biomarkers for delayed graft function following kidney transplantation. *Am. J. Transplant.* 2006; 6: 1639-1645.

[58] Zhang P, Rothblum L, Han WK, Blasick T, Potdar S, Bonventre JV. Kidney injury molecule-1 expression in transplant biopsies is a sensitive measure of cell injury. *Kidney Int.* 2008; 73: 608-614.

[59] Mehta RL, Kellum JA, Shah SV, Molitoris BA, Ronco C, Warnock DG, Levin A; Acute Kidney Injury Network. Acute Kidney Injury Network: report of an initiative to improve outcomes in acute kidney injury. *Crit. Care.* 2007; 11: R31.

[60] Levy EM, Viscoli CM, Horwitz RI. The effect of acute renal failure on mortality. A cohort analysis. *JAMA* 1996; 275: 1489-1494.

[61] Lassnigg A, Schmidlin D, Mouhieddine M, Bachmann LM, Druml W, Bauer P, Hiesmayr M. Minimal changes of serum creatinine predict prognosis in patients after cardiothoracic surgery: A prospective cohort study. *J. Am. Soc. Nephrol.* 2004; 15: 1597-1605.

[62] Barrantes F, Feng Y, Ivanov O, Yalamanchili HB, Patel J, Buenafe X, Cheng V, Dijeh S, Amoateng-Adjepong Y, Manthous CA. Acute kidney injury predicts outcomes of non-critically ill patients. *Mayo Clin. Proc.* 2009; 84: 410-416.

[63] Barrantes F, Tian J, Vazquez R, Amoateng-Adjepong Y, Manthous CA. Acute kidney injury criteria predict outcomes of critically ill patients. *Crit. Care Med.* 2008; 36: 1397-1403.

[64] Bagshaw SM, George C, Bellomo R, for the ANZICS Database Management Committee. A comparison of the RIFLE and AKIN criteria for acute kidney injury in critically ill patients. *Nephrol. Dial. Transplant.* 2008; 23: 1569-1574.

[65] Joannidis M, Metnitz B, Bauer P, Schusterschitz N, Moreno R, Druml W, Metnitz PG. Acute kidney injury in critically ill patients classified by AKIN versus RIFLE using the SAPS 3 database. *Intensive Care Med.* 2009; 35:1692-1702.

[66] Kellum JA, Bellomo R, Ronco C. Classification of acute kidney injury using RIFLE: What's the purpose? *Crit. Care Med.* 2007; 35: 1983-1984.

[67] Cruz DN, Ricci Z, Ronco C. Clinical review: RIFLE and AKIN - time for reappraisal. *Crit. Care.* 2009; 13: 211.

In: Acute Kidney Injury: Causes, Diagnosis and Treatments   ISBN: 978-1-61209-790-9
Editor: Jonathan D. Mendoza, pp. 19-35   © 2011 Nova Science Publishers, Inc.

Chapter II

Acute Renal Failure in the Newborn (NB)

Nilzete Liberato Bresolin
Federal University of Santa Catarina, Brazil

Abstract

Despite advances in neonatal and perinatal medicine the assessment of the renal function of newborns remains a major challenge. The unique features of neonates defy the ability to understand and define acute kidney injury (AKI) in this age group. The studies on the subject are scarce and mostly based on a small numbers of patients and performed in single centers. Up until now, observational studies suggest that critically ill neonates have high rates of AKI with a guarded prognosis. Moreover, newborns with AKI can develop a renal function impairment, proteinuria and hypertension requiring long term monitoring. Appropriate evaluation of renal function represents the first step towards the recognition and early treatment of AKI (elimination of risk factors) and a change in the short and long-term prognosis of critically ill newborns.

Keywords: Renal function, newborn, assessment.

Introduction

The production of urine, the major component of amniotic fluid in the second half of pregnancy, is an important function of the fetal kidneys in intrauterine life. Thus, when failure occurs to the fetal renal function due to the inability to produce urine (intrinsic renal failure or renal malformation) or due to the inability to eliminate it (obstructive uropathy) oligohydramnios may occur that, if uncorrected, will result in a Potter's syndrome, with a high early postnatal mortality.[1] On the other hand, from the moment that the umbilical cord is clamped and cut, several physiological mechanisms are rapidly activated to ensure the survival of the newborn (NB). Regarding renal function, newborns have physiological and possible anatomic characteristics that suggest immaturity of this system. Such elements of immaturity, of course, will be exacerbated in premature newborns. Knowing them may help prevent the development of AKI in this age. The more relevant of the immature kidney functions are as follow:

- Low glomerular filtration rate (GFR) due to low renal blood flow and high intrarenal vascular resistance.
- Limited capacity to concentrate urine due to low concentration of interstitial medullary, decreased responsiveness to antidiuretic hormone (ADH), short loops of Henle and interference with prostaglandins.
- Decreased ability of tubular sodium reabsorption due to lower response to aldosterone contributing to increased risk of hyperkalemia in these patients.[1]
- Moreover, since nephrogenesis continues up until 34-35 weeks of gestation, hypoxic-ischemic or toxic damage to the kidney in development of preterm newborns (PTNB) may result in AKI and long-term complications associated with the potential interruption of nephrogenesis.[2]

For all these factors the incidence of acute kidney injury (AKI) in the neonatal period is greater than in later childhood, although the exact number remains undetermined due to the lack of common diagnostic criteria, existence of cases characterized by transient oliguria that were never recognized, as well as cases of nonoliguric AKI, even the severe cases, often not diagnosed.[3,4,5]

In a recent publication Ringer[3] reaffirms the difficulty of defining AKI in newborns based on specific values of creatinine because of the following reasons: serum creatinine levels in the NB after birth reflected maternal creatinine and not the renal function of the NB; normal values of creatinine depends on the gestational and postnatal age of the child. In addition, creatinine reflects muscle mass, and both in childhood and in adulthood the values depend on age, sex, clinical conditions (e.g. fever) and volume distribution.[6,7] The prognosis for the NB with AKI is variable and dependent on comorbidities and complications of other organs, as well as the underlying disease that resulted in AKI.[1,3,8] The mortality rate can be as high as 61% in patients with multiple organ dysfunction syndrome (MODS) and, recently, authors have shown that renal damage has an independent impact on the survival of newborns even after correcting for comorbidities, complications and disease severity.[1,3,9]

Furthermore, there is a substantial risk of future renal damage independent of the etiology and clinical and experimental studies have called attention to the importance of monitoring patients diagnosed with AKI.[2,4,10] Several authors point to the need for routine monitoring of the renal function, proteinuria and hypertension even when the creatinine presents normal values for the child's age at discharge, and emphasize that change in any of these items may take years to appear.[2,4,5,6,10,11,12] Early diagnosis and prompt institution of appropriate treatment for each clinical situation may change the course and severity of renal impairment, and influence towards the morbidity and mortality rates of patients in the acute phase and in later life. In this contest, factors related to the renal function of newborns, as well as new diagnostic criteria and monitoring of AKI in the neonatal period will be further discussed.

Characteristics of the Kidney in the Newborn

The kidney of the newborn is particularly prone to the development of AKI due to working with very low GFR, which is maintained by a delicate balance between vasoconstrictor and vasodilator forces. Although this GFR is sufficient to maintain growth and development under normal conditions, these low values limit the postnatal functional adaptation to stress (endogenous and exogenous), especially in newborn babies of very low birth weight (VLBW) because of prematurity or intrauterine growth restriction.[3,13] Moreover, there is the influence of other factors including low systemic blood pressure, high renal vascular resistance and low renal blood flow.

In newborns the renal blood flow is equivalent to 3 to 7% of cardiac output whereas in adults it is equivalent to 25% of cardiac output. At birth there is a loss of placental blood flow and gradual increase of renal blood flow reaching adult levels by the age of 2 years.[3,13] The fact that nephrogenesis is maintained until 34 to 35 weeks of gestation and that the extrauterine environment does not seem to be ideal for the glomerular development is particularly important.[5,8] This negative effect may be exacerbated in patients with AKI.[5,8] Thus, hypoxic/ischemic and toxic insults to the developing kidney in a PTNB can result in not only AKI but also in long-term complications associated with potential interruption of nephrogenesis. Besides, there is evidence that the PTNB are at an increased risk of hypertension, chronic kidney disease and metabolic syndrome.[5,8,10] Given this predisposition to renal impairment, the early identification and, where possible, elimination of predisposing factors is essential to preserve the renal function of newborns.[2,3]

Acute Renal Impairment in Newborns

Advances in neonatal and perinatal medicine have improved the survival rate of critically ill newborns; however, the morbidity and mortality rates are still significant. Ill newborns are at risk of developing AKI because they are commonly exposed to nephrotoxic medications and infectious conditions that can result in MODS. [8] AKI is a complex disorder with clinical manifestations ranging from mild renal dysfunction to severe conditions of acute anuric renal failure. In NB 60 to 90% of cases of AKI are pre-renal in origin, although it is understood now that genetic factors may predispose some newborns to develop AKI.[3,14,15,16] The majority of pre-renal causes is recoverable with proper handling, however, in the long term, some patients can develop renal impairment.[3,9,16]

The primary causes of renal failure represented by congenital renal diseases such as autosomal dominant or recessive polycystic kidney disease and bilateral renal hypoplasia anomaly are less frequent (11%) and post renal which account for 3% of all cases of AKI result from obstruction in a solitary kidney, bilateral ureteral obstruction, urethral obstruction (posterior urethral valve), or neurogenic bladder caused by myelomeningocele and etc.[1] It is necessary to remember that in newborns AKI may have a prenatal onset in congenital diseases like renal dysplasia with or without obstructive uropathy and in genetic diseases such as recessive polycystic kidney disease or due to maternal use of drugs, such as converting enzyme inhibitors (ACEi), angiotensin II receptor blockers (ARBs), antibiotics, non-steroidal anti-inflammatory drugs (NSAIDs) and illicit drugs.[1,3,13,16] However, as with older children AKI is commonly acquired in the postnatal period in-hospital due to hypoxic-ischemic or nephrotoxic insults (aminoglycosides, vancomycin, amphotericin and administration of NSAIDs for closure of patent ductus arteriovenous), sepsis and post cardiac surgery.[1,3,8,16,17.18]

The majority of newborns who receive indomethacin present impaired renal function, which is usually reversible if there is no associated nephrotoxic factors. Vascular lesions (renal artery or renal vein thrombosis) can also result in AKI if bilateral or if they occur in a solitary kidney. In addition, there are also interstitial nephritis and renal impairment secondary to an infectious condition (pyelonephritis, sepsis, syphilis, toxoplasmosis, and obstructive fungus ball secondary to candidiasis). [13]

Physiopathology

The reduction in renal plasma flow secondary to hypovolemia or impairment of cardiac output is the marker of pre-renal lesion. The adequate correction of these disturbances often allows a complete recovery of renal hypoperfusion and restoration of its function. On the other hand, delays in recognizing and treating these conditions may result in impairment of renal vascular responses and a decreased renal plasma flow even after the correction of volemia.[3,16]

In healthy newborns (in spite of the systemic blood pressure and renal blood flow normally low), blood flow and renal perfusion can be maintained even in the presence of the reduction of systemic blood pressure. The mechanism of self-regulation to maintain renal blood flow occurs by dilation of afferent arterioles and constriction of efferent arterioles. This mechanism results from the increased secretion of catecholamines (triggered by reduced renal perfusion) which causes generation of prostacyclin and prostaglandin vasodilators and can be affected by many drugs. Catecholamines also activate the renin-angiotensin-aldosterone system (RAAS), which mediates the efferent vasoconstriction. However, if there is a contraction of volemia, a decrease of the ability to self-regulate occurs placing the newborn at high risk of developing AKI.[3]

It should also be noted that the glomerular filtration depends on the difference between the transcapillary hydrostatic pressure and pressure in the proximal tubule.[19] Studies show that when hypotension is intense enough to fall below the capacity for self-regulation, hypofiltration and decreased renal function occur.[19]

The physiologic immaturity may accentuate the impact of reducing the transcapillary hydrostatic pressure making it more important than hypovolemia or decreased cardiac output in the reduction of GFR. The transcapillary pressure also depends on the hydrostatic pressure in the proximal tubule.

In situations of tubular lesion with cell death and rupture of the membrane, tubular obstruction may occur and also an increase in intratubular pressure with consequent decrease in transcapillary pressure and in glomerular filtration. There could still be loss or damage to intracellular junctions with creatinine leaks from the tubule back into the circulation from peritubular capillaries.[3] The alterations in properties of the glomerular membrane can also be important during the gestational maturation.[3]

Definition of AKI

Despite the high incidence of AKI in adults, neonates and older children, until recently, the lack of universal definition limited the ability to compare studies, predict a clinical course and consequently improve its prognosis.[4,8,16] Against this background, the Acute Dialysis Quality Initiative (ADQI) held the Second International Consensus Conference in May 2002 in the city of Vicenza.[20] AQDI, was formed in early 2000 and was composed of nephrologists and intensivists, including pediatric representation. The group objectively scrutinized available AKI data and classified it as to scientific merit. From this analysis, criteria for AKI in adults was proposed and defined. These criteria are known as RIFLE criteria (Risk of dysfunction, Injury to the kidney, Failure of kidney function, Loss of kidney function, end-stage renal disease).[20] The findings were published in 2004 and are currently being validated in the scientific community through various studies that reference it.[18] RIFLE criteria define three grades of severity of AKI - Risk (class R), Injury (class I) and Failure (class F) - and two classes of evolution (Loss - Class L - and End-Stage - Class E).[20] In the first three categories, the RIFLE criteria standardize the definition of AKI by stratification of patients according to changes in the levels of serum creatinine and urinary output from baseline levels. Loss of renal function, and the end-stage renal disease define two clinical categories based on time evolution of renal replacement therapy (RRT) required after the start of insult.[20] Recently Akcan-Arikan et al. [21] developed a modified version of RIFLE for pediatric patients (pRIFLE). The pRIFLE proposed criteria are based on reducing the estimated creatinine clearance (eCCL) and urine output, and its details are summarized in Table 1. [21] However, so far we found only one study involving critically ill neonates and our service is initiating a protocol for analysis of the RIFLE criteria in newborns.[22] Publications of pediatric studies based on the pRIFLE criteria begin to open up the possibility of inter-center comparisons of AKI cases.[16,21,23,24]

Diagnosis of AKI: Clinical and Laboratorial Aspects

As in most cases the signs and symptoms of AKI are nonspecific there is a need for a high degree of clinical suspicion in patients at risk. Newborns, due to renal immaturity, are considered high-risk patients. The diagnosis, as in other diseases, must be founded on history, physical examination and laboratory data and imaging, valuing information on predisposing factors (hemodynamic alterations, hypoxic-ischemic disorders, and use of nephrotoxic agents), increased renal size, abdominal mass or a palpable bladder.

Furthermore, although the presence of oliguria (defined as urine output less than 0.5ml/Kg/hour for 8 to 12 hours) serves as an alert to the possibility of AKI, it is not present in many patients, and especially the VLBW newborns and the extremely low birth weight newborns often present AKI with a normal or increased urine output.[1,3,13,25] On the other hand, it should be noted that the onset of urination may take up to 24 hours in some normal newborns. And the VLBW newborns may have phases of transient oliguria that spontaneously revert.[25]

Table 1. Pediatric RIFLE criteria (pRIFLE)[21]

	Estimated creatinine clearance (eCCL)	Urine output
Risk	eCCL decrease by 25%	<0.5 ml/(kg h) for 8 h
Injury	eCCL decrease by 50%	<0.5 ml/(kg h) for 16 h
Failure	eCCL decrease by 75% or eCCL <35 ml/min/1.73 m²	<0.5 ml/(kg h) for 24 h ou anuric for 12 h
Lost	Persistent failure >4 weeks	
End-stage	End-stage renal disease (Persistent >3months)	

Since situations that can cause pre-renal AKI can also result in AKI itself (in most cases, acute tubular necrosis) there is a need for an early diagnosis to establish the appropriate treatment and prevent the evolution.[3,16] The cases of pre-renal AKI require, in addition to specific measures aimed at the underlying disease, maintenance of volemia, cardiac output, blood pressure and, whenever possible, replace nephrotoxic agents by non- nephrotoxic agents. Where this is not possible a drug dosage adjustment is recommended according to the creatinine clearance.[1,13] The cases of ATN after restoration of volemia and institution of measures to treat the underlying disease, need adequacy of drinking water, which can be restrictive (replacement of insensible losses or less associated with diuresis and abnormal losses) until the diuretic response is noted or whether a RRT is indicated.[25] Moreover, the same cautions mentioned above in relation to nephrotoxic agents with special attention to patients in RRT must be taken, since there are dialyzable and other non-dialyzable drugs.[1,3] In cases with impairment of volemia the fluid deficit can be corrected with a bolus of saline solution of 10 to 20 ml/kg intravenously. In cases of pre-renal AKI, diuresis can be seen in a few hours. After correction of volemia, if there was no diuretic response, furosemide may be administered at 1mg/kg and wait for a diuresis of 1ml/kg/hour. If there is no diuresis the hypothesis of AKI is then established.[25] In addition to the situations described above, many drugs can cause nephrotoxicity.[3,16,26] Medications commonly associated with AKI, in part due to tubular impairment, include aminoglycosides, contrast media, amphotericin, chemotherapeutic agents (ifosfamide and cisplatin), acyclovir and acetominofen.[16] Exemplifying, the nephrotoxicity of aminoglycosides is characterized by non-oliguric AKI and minimal urinary abnormalities and therefore requires a high degree of suspicion and laboratorial control for the diagnosis. In this case the nephrotoxicity is related to the dose, dosing interval, duration of antibiotic therapy and renal function prior to initiation of therapy with aminoglycosides.[3,16] Although changes in glomerular ultrastructure may also occur, it is more commonly believed that there is a tubular injury due to dysfunction of lysosomes of proximal tubules, reversible with discontinuation of the drug.[16] However, it should be noted that even after discontinuation of the aminoglycoside there may be an increase of serum creatinine (for several days) by persistence of tubular injury associated with the high drug concentration at the parenchymal levels.[16] Although the process is reversible AKI is associated with rising costs, longer hospitalization and higher mortality rates clearly justify prevention efforts.[3,8,9,21,23,24,26] In a recent review Ringer[3] highlights that, similar to what occurs in adults, administration of aminoglycosides once daily has also become standard practice in neonates. In patients at risk for AKI, it is recommended, whenever possible, the use of alternative antimicrobials.[16,27] Failing this option, the renal function should be accessed concurrently with daily monitoring of the drug serum levels. Another agent commonly used and potentially nephrotoxic is amphotericin.[16,27] In this case, the new liposomal formulations should be opted for, as they, infrequently, cause nephrotoxicity in the NB.[3] Compared to vancomycin, whose mechanism of nephrotoxicity remains unknown, great care should be taken to the synergistic nephrotoxic action of the combination with aminoglycosides, and whenever possible, alternative agents should be used. Monitoring the serum levels is fundamental in patients using vancomycin.[1,27] On the other hand, the non-steroidal anti-inflammatory drugs (NSAIDs) used to treat patent ductus arteriosus with hemodynamic impairment may aggravate the impairment of renal disease. As previously mentioned, the renal function of the newborn is kept through self-regulatory mechanisms involving dilation of afferent and efferent arteriolar constriction (which are prostaglandin-dependent). NSAIDs block prostaglandin synthesis and may reduce GFR, the urinary output causing excess of free water and metabolic disorders.[3] The inhibitors of angiotensin converting enzyme (ACE) can also impair the autoregulation of renal blood flow by blocking vasoconstriction in the efferent arteriole and should be used cautiously in newborns. Both NSAIDs and ACE inhibitors when used by the mother during pregnancy may have an impact on the fetal renal function and on the NB.[3] In the context of nephrotoxicity, it must be remembered that haemolysis and rhabdomyolysis, regardless of cause, could result in hemoglobinuria or myoglobinuria and induce renal tubular lesion associated with vasoconstriction, precipitation of pigment in the tubular lumen and oxidative stress induced by heme-protein.[3,16] Also in relation to clinical cases of AKI there is an important consideration regarding patients after cardiac surgery; as at least two clinical forms of AKI can be recognized in these patients:[21,22]

- Early AKI that occurs in the postoperative period and is more commonly related to the surgical procedure (by cardiopulmonary bypass or low output syndrome by transient left ventricular dysfunction, secondary to the release of free oxygen radicals in response to induction of inflammatory condition), to the time of prolonged cardiopulmonary bypass (CPB) or to the state of intraoperative hypotension.
- Late AKI that occurs a few days after surgery and may result from the use of nephrotoxic agents, hemodynamic disorders, sepsis and MODS.

Having made the above considerations, the definitive diagnosis of AKI which is problematic at any age will now be discussed, because it is based on two functional abnormalities: changes in serum creatinine levels (a marker of GFR) and oliguria (that has been previously discussed).[8] Both functional abnormalities are a consequence of the lesion and no markers of the lesion itself.[8] Recently Ringer[3] reaffirmed the difficulty of diagnosing AKI in the neonate period based on specific values of creatinine. The serum concentrations of creatinine in the first days after birth reflect the maternal creatinine and not the newborn's renal function.[3,8] It is also important the fact that the normal nephrogenesis begins with 8 weeks of gestation and continues until 34 - 35 weeks of gestation, when the number of nephrons of 1.6 million to 2.4 million approaches the number of adults. So, depending on the degree of prematurity of the NB, GFR increases from 10 to 20ml/min/1.73m² body surface during the first week of life with 30 to 40 ml/min/m² around the second week after birth, concomitant with changes in renal blood flow. Recently, Schwartz et al[28] demonstrated that GFR increases significantly during the first months of life. Overall, GFR in TNB and PNB is very low and there is a great variation in the distribution of normal values of creatinine, which vary greatly depending on the degree of prematurity and age of the patient (Tables 2, 3 and 4).[3,8,28,29,30,31,32,33] As shown in Tables 2, 3 and 4 creatinine values depend on the gestational age, and these are higher in more immature and postnatal ages.[3,28,29,30,31,32,33] In TNB concentrations usually increase during the first 24 to 36 hours after birth, subsequently decrease and stabilize at around 0.5 mg/dl around the fifth day of life.[3] In premature newborns the peak occurs between 2 and 3 days after birth and stabilize around the sixth day of life. These variations make it difficult to use single values for creatinine to diagnose AKI, and therefore often we use the daily elevations of serum levels (or absence of levels reduction observed at birth) and, more recently, according to the pRIFLE criteria, reduction of creatinine clearance or urine output.[3,5,20,21] In practical terms, GFR can be estimated using the Schwartz formula that uses serum creatinine concentration in mg/dl, the patient's height in cm and a constant K related to body mass and creatinine urinary excretion which can be applied to the TNB and PNB.[28,33]

In premature newborns: Estimated GFR (mL/min/1.73m²): $\dfrac{0.33 \text{ X height (cm)}}{\text{serum creatinine (mg/dl)}}$

In full-term newborns: Estimated GFR (mL/min/1.73m²): $\dfrac{0.45 \text{ X height (cm)}}{\text{serum creatinine (mg/dl)}}$

Creatinine, as previously mentioned, is a metabolic product of creatine and phosphocreatine muscle and is related to muscle mass of each patient.[7,8] Studies in adults and children showed that serum creatinine levels also vary with age, sex, meat content of the person's diet, nutritional state, catabolic state, presence of liver disease and volume of distribution (which can be suddenly increased during the fluid resuscitation of seriously ill patient).[34] There are also conditions that increase creatinine production (muscle trauma, fever, and immobilization) and conditions that decrease its production (liver disease, reduced muscle mass) that must be considered in the interpretation of creatinine serum levels.[34] It should also be highlighted that recent studies have questioned the sensitivity of creatinine in the initial diagnosis of AKI and that even small changes in serum levels during the first 48 hours after cardiac surgery, are associated with significant increase in mortality.[35] This last observation may reflect the fact that the serum creatinine concentration may not change until 25 to 50% of renal function has been lost and therefore it may take days before an increase of its levels occurs.[8]

Table 2. Plasma creatinine values at birth[3]

Gestacional age (weeks)	Creatinine mg/dl
23 a 26	0.77 a 1.05
27 a 29	0.76 a 1.02
30 a 32	0.70 a 0.80
33 a 45	0.77 a 0.90

Adapted from: Ringer AS. Acute renal failure in the neonate. NeoReviews. 2010;11;e243-e251.

Table 3. Plasma Creatinine Values in Term and Preterm Infants (mean ± SD)[29,30,31]

Age (d)	<28wk	28-32wk	32-37wk	>37wk
3	1.05±0.27	0.88±0.25	0.78±0.22	0.75±0.2
7	0.95±0.36	0.94±0.37	0.77±0.48	0.56±0.4
14	0.81±0.26	0.78±0.36	0.62±0.4	0.43±0.25
28	0.66±0.28	0.59±0.38	0.40±0.28	0.34±0.2

Adapted from Rudd PT Huges EA, Placzek MM. Reference ranges for plasma creatinine during the first month of life. Arch Dis Child 1983;58:212-5.[30] Van den AnKer JN, de Groot R, Broerse HM. Assesment of glomerular filtration rate in preterm infants by serum creatinine: Comparison with insulin clearance. Pediatrics 1995;96:1156-58.[31]

Table 4. Glomerular Filtration Rate (ml/min/1.73m^2) in Newborn [32]

G A (weeks)	CCl	Post-Natal Age		
		1^a week	2^a week	3^a week
25 a 28	ClCr corrigido	5.6 – 16.4	9.3 – 21.7	25.9 – 68.9
29 a 37	ClCr corrigido	9.7 – 20.9	14.9 – 42.5	33.0 – 70.0
38 a 42	ClCr corrigido	25.8 – 54.5	41.0 – 90.6	74.0 – 117.4

Adapted from Schwartz JG, Brian LP, Spitzer A. The use of plasma creatinine concentration for estimating glomerular filtration rate in infants, children and adolescents. Pediatr Clin North Am. 1987; 34: 571-90.[32]
GA: gestacional age CCl: creatinine clearance

Another important point is that different methods for measuring levels of creatinine (Jaffé x enzymatic) produce different values. When the determination is performed using the Jaffe method elevated serum levels of bilirubin can cause artificial reduction of creatinine, and certain drugs such as cephalosporin can produce artificial elevation of these valores.[8] Specifically, in relation to the interference of bilirubin with the method of Jaffe, it should be remembered that PNB have normal levels of bilirubin at birth which increase during the first days of life and return to normal after a few weeks.[8] In practical terms, even if there are questions for the adequacy of the dosage of drugs administered to patients with impaired renal function, tables are employed that suggest dosage adjustments from the estimated creatinine clearance.[27,36] These adjustments are particularly important for the adequacy of renal elimination drugs whose inadequate administration could cause nephrotoxicity and ototoxicity.[3] Obviously, since it uses the serum creatinine to assess GFR, the results are subject to all the limitations described above related to creatinine. Serum urea, generated from the catabolism of amino acids in the liver, is freely filtered by the glomerulus. However, unlike creatinine, it suffers 40-50% of reabsorption in the proximal tubule or in the medullary collecting tubule. Its values are less useful than the creatinine to monitor renal function because the serum levels suffer influence from hypercatabolism, amount of protein in the diet, gastrointestinal bleeding and tubular reabsorption that may be elevated in renal hypoperfusion states.[34]

Table 5. Urine Indices in Prerenal and Intrinsec Renal Failure [3]

	Urine Osmolality (mOsm/L)	Urine sodium (mEq/L)	FENa (%)
Prerenal (child)	400-500	<10-20	< 1.0
Prerenal (newborn and preterm)	> 350	< 20-30	< 2.5
AKI (ATN)	< 350	> 30-40	>2.0

Adapted from: Ringer AS. Acute renal failure in the neonate. NeoReviews. 2010;11;e243-e251.
FENa: fractional excretion of sodium; ATN (acute tubular necrosis)

An elevation of urea can also be observed, disproportionate to the increase in creatinine in the following situations: use of corticosteroids, the use of tetracycline or against any inflammatory stimulus that increases the synthesis of urea.[34] Regarding urinalysis, in cases of AKI itself, granular cylinders and proteinuria in varying degrees can be observed. Due to the loss of ability to retain water and sodium, with decreased ability to conserve sodium and, consequently, decreased urinary osmolality, increased urinary sodium and increased fractional excretion of sodium (FENa).[16] These indices, as well as in older patients, can help differentiate between prerenal AKI and AKI itself caused by ATN.[3] (Table 5). However, it is stressed that, especially in premature newborns due to renal tubular immaturity, the usefulness of these indices is limited.[3] In addition, they must be obtained before the administration of loop diuretics or thiazides, and sympathomimetic amines which, for causing natriuresis, interfere with results.[1,13] In imaging investigation ultrasonography (USG) and perfusion analysis of the renal artery by Doppler is useful in evaluating kidneys with renal function impairment or with no renal function. A MAG3 (Mercaptoacetyl triglycerin) renal scintigraphy can be performed soon after birth.[25] The MAG3 Renal scintigraphy with the USG, provide information about the urinary tract (size, shape, dilation, obstruction, masses) on the renal parenchyma (cysts, increased echogenicity and loss of corticomedullary differentiation in the ATN, renal atrophy, etc.) and on the permeability of the renal vessels.[13,25] The voiding cystourethrography helps in the diagnosis of post-renal causes of AKI.[25] The excretory urogram, due to contrast nephrotoxicity, may aggravate AKI and should be avoided.

New Biomarkers

As previously reported, early changes in renal function as measured by small changes in serum creatinine levels may reflect significant renal insults and be associated with high morbidity and mortality.[16,21,23,24,35] This occurs because the concentration of creatinine is considered by many authors, an insensitive and late marker of the impairment of renal function.[6,34,35] So are several recent studies focused on the search for new (and earlier) biomarkers of renal impairment.[8,16, 37] Among them, the following are highlighted: the serum and urine levels of neutrophil gelatinase associated lipocalin (NGAL), interleukin 18 (IL-18), the kidney injury molecule-1 (KIM-1) and serum cystatin.[8,38] NGAL presents a significant expression after renal ischemia. Its serum and urine levels are elevated in human models of AKI, including newborns in post-surgery with cardiopulmonary bypass, as well as in the critically ill pediatric population.[8,37,38] Levels of IL-18 are elevated in adults with ischemic AKI, in newborns with AKI after cardiopulmonary bypass and in children with AKI without sepsis but not in children with sepsis and AKI. This fact (IL-18 is not elevated in children with sepsis and AKI) justifies the need for new biomarkers to be tested in different populations and different clinical situations.[8,38] In relation to KIM-1, the advantage is that its expression is limited to the disease or renal impairment and there is no description of other systemic sources. However, its levels may be influenced by nephrotoxins and by various nephropathies.[38] Cystatin C is a protein of low molecular weight produced at a constant rate by all nucleated cells, removed from circulation by glomerular filtration only, completely resorbed and not secreted by tubular cells. It has been shown in several studies as a more sensitive marker of renal function than creatinine.[38,39,40] Zappitelli [39] affirms in a recent review that, in studies of post-cardiac surgery with cardiopulmonary bypass (in adults and children), cystatin C may rise 1 to 2 days before the increase in creatinine in patients with AKI. In the neonatal period, Armangil et a [41] affirm that as cystatin C does not cross the placenta, its values in neonates reflect only their GFR and not the mother's GFR, as is the case with creatinine. Notwithstanding these considerations, however, there are limitations on the measurement of cystatin C to be registered and which include the high costs and the fact that they are not easily available. There are also controversial views on possible factors influencing its levels. Andersen TB e cols [42] also affirm that although the sensitivity of cystatin C to detect reduced GFR appears to be superior to creatinine, especially in children with small muscle mass, there is a need for further studies to evaluate the influence of C-reactive protein levels, corticoids, thyroid dysfunction and decompensated diabetes for the determination of cystatin C. Obviously, the sensitivity and specificity of these biomarkers should be validated in multicenter clinical trials. Anyway, the availability of a panel of biomarkers will revolutionize the care of critically ill patients, because by enabling the diagnosis of AKI occurrence in a few hours after the insult, they will ensure a differentiated approach to them.

Suggested Intervals for the Control of Renal Function

Depending on the patient's clinical condition and the medicines that are being used, a daily control of renal function may be necessary. If there is an impairment of renal function, whenever possible, the daily serum levels of aminoglycosides and vancomycin should be requested for a dose adjustment according to creatinine clearances and in patients on a dialysis procedure, in accordance with the elimination or not of the drug through the dialysis method.[36]

Handling the IRA in the NB

After those considerations on etiology, pathophysiology, and diagnosis; we will now move to the handling, itself, of AKI in the NB. As discussed earlier, the handling should start with the prevention of renal lesion based on the identification of patients at risk and eliminate, where possible, predisposing factors, in addition to treating the underlying disease and maintaining homeostasis. These measures aim at limiting or preventing new renal lesions. Patients at risk are: anoxiated by pre-natal or post-natal problems, children of mothers who used drugs (e.g. NSAIDs, ACE inhibitors) the shocked ones of any etiology, drug users of drugs such as NSAIDs, ACE inhibitors, aminoglycosides, vancomycin, amphotericin; those who underwent catheterization of umbilical vessels, patients with massive hemolysis that may evolve with hemoglobinuria, and the patients with rhabdomyolysis secondary to infectious or metabolic disturbances (phosphorus, potassium, calcium or sodium disorders), and can change with myoglobinuria which, as well as hemoglobinuria, can be toxic to tubular cells and cause renal vasoconstriction resulting in renal lesion.[3,4,16] In these patients, we must eliminate the predisposing factors from the restoration of hydroelectrolytic homeostasis, adequacy of oxygenation, replacement or adjustment of doses of nephrotoxic drugs according to creatinine clearance, urine alkalinization, aggressive hydration and use of diuretics (in cases of hemoglobinuria or myoglobinuria that respond to diuresis).[5] The treatment of ARF itself can be carried out with conservative measures and dialysis. Moreover, the conservative treatment should include measures to maintain homeostasis (balance of supply of oxygen, optimization of cardiac output and supply of fluids according to volume state and age of the patient, correction of hydroelectrolyte and acid-base disturbances), adequacy of nutritional support to patient needs. Regarding the use of furosemide which does not seem to interfere with the course of the AKI established, most authors agree that its use is justified, for maintaining water homeostasis and elimination of potassium in patients who respond to its use with diuresis.[16] Moreover, it has the advantage of inhibiting the mechanism of counter-current level of the ascending limb of Henle's loops (AAH) and thus reduce the consumption of oxygen in the external renal medulla (already damaged tubules with low supply of oxygen).[16] With the increase of the tubular urine flow, the risk of tubular obstruction by cellular debris or debris is minimized. On the other hand, disadvantages include ototoxicity, nephrotoxicity mainly by the use in bolus and in high doses.[16,43] A persistent patent ductus arteriosus may also occur due to a furosemide-induced stimulation of prostaglandin E_2, renal calcification risk (by increasing the elimination of calcium in urine), and also diuretic resistance by the drug's chronic use.[43] A diuretic resistance should be suspected in patients with chronic use of drugs in which diuretic response decreases without any change in renal function or in the supply of fluids.[43] This can be treated with prior administration of low doses of thiazide in 0.5 to 1 hour. This situation results from hypertrophy of the distal tubule cells to compensate for the high supply of sodium in this tubular segment secondary to the inhibition of the counter-current mechanism due to the prolonged use of the diuretic and can be treated with a combination of thiazide diuretics, which are also indicated to prevent nephrocalcinosis.[43]

Regarding whether the mode of administration should be by bolus or continuous infusion, studies show that bolus infusion has greater neuroendocrine stimulation and that the continuous infusion promotes maintenance of diuresis with less ototoxicity in relation to the conventional use of intermittent bolus. It should be observed that furosemide is contraindicated in situations of anuria secondary to volume depletion and hepatic coma.[43] Regarding the use of dopamine in the NB with AKI most authors agree that hypotensive newborns, unresponsive to fluid administration, require the use of vasoactive and inotropic drugs for the adequacy of cardiac output and renal blood flow. However, although dopamine actually increases cardiac output and renal blood flow promoting vasodilation and is also able to improve urinary output with increased natriuresis, it has also side effects that include an increased risk of arrhythmia, development of intrapulmonary shunt and impaired responses to T lymphocytes.[16] Meta-analysis concluded that its use for the treatment and prevention of AKI is not justified based on current clinical evidence.[44] It is worth mentioning here that fenoldopan, a selective dopaminergic agonist for type 1 receptors (DA-1), short-acting, which reduces vascular resistance and causes increased renal blood flow, has been the subject of several studies. A recently published meta-analysis[45] concluded that it reduces the incidence of AKI, reduces the need for renal replacement therapy (RRT), and the period of stay in ICU as well as the mortality rate. The pediatric experience with fenoldopan is scarce but promising.[46]

In relation to nutritional support, it is important to remember that protein restriction does not apply to severely ill newborns due not only to the risk of the loss of body mass (due to the common association with hypercatabolism), but also to the risk of organ dysfunction and immune deficiency. Thus, in the cases where there is difficulty in maintaining the water balance RRT should be indicated to ensure an adequate nutritional support. In choosing the route of administration, if the gastrointestinal tract is intact and functioning, an enteral nutrition should be chosen. The option must be breast milk or formulas with a low renal solute and phosphorus content. An adequate energy supply should be offered aiming at promoting anabolism and preventing catabolism, which could aggravate metabolic disorders, such as hyperphosphatemia, hyperkalemia and acidosis.[47] If oral feeding is not tolerated, administer parenteral nutrition with at least 50Kcal/Kg/day, 1 to 2 grams of protein/kg/day (energy intake is rarely achieved in an oliguric NB). Regarding the type of amino acids, although there was controversy, currently the suggestion is that essential and nonessential amino acids be administered because these often become compulsorily essential.

In addition to the conservative treatment, the handling of AKI also often requires the RRT that can be divided into standard methods: peritoneal dialysis (PD) and intermittent hemodialysis (IH) and into continuous methods: hemofiltration (HF) and associated techniques: hemodiafiltration and more recently: prolonged hemodialysis. The RRT will be indicated more by clinical parameters than laboratorial parameters: in situations of failure of the conservative treatment (severe metabolic acidosis, a life-threatening hyperkalemia, fluid overload, symptomatic hyperuricaemia), difficulty in the adequacy of nutritional support or in cases of AKI and poor general health.[48,49] As for the choice of method, it should be noted that the preference for HF has increased among pediatric nephrologists compared with PD except for NN and small infants. The PD remains the method of choice for newborns in several countries due to technical ease, low cost, and greater relationship between the peritoneal surface and body surface.[1,9]

Among the undesirable effects of PD are increased intra-abdominal pressure which may result in leakage and hernias, reduction of venous return and cardiac output by up to 25% of its normal values and reduced pulmonary functional residual capacity by diaphragmatic elevation. The latter can be deleterious for patients with AKI and the risk of hypoxemia may in some cases be balanced with baths with volumes of 5 to 10ml/Kg.[13,48] The contraindications, often relative, include: necrotizing enterocolitis, severe or complicated, recent abdominal surgery (<48 hours), abdominal wall defects, hemorrhagic diathesis, ventricle-peritoneal shunt.[13]

In these cases there is the option of the HI or continuous methods. The HI allows a rapid correction of metabolic abnormalities (particularly important in those disorders associated with hyperammonemia in urea cycle disorders) and rapid correction of hypervolemia. Disadvantages include the need for heparinization, highly purified water and specialized technical staff. Contraindications are hemodynamic instability and severe hemorrhage. [48] The continuous methods, in turn, have the following advantages: solute clearance and continuous ultrafiltration, mimicking the function of the kidney, particularly useful in hypervolemic newborns with acute pulmonary edema, requiring parenteral nutrition support and drugs.[48] The patient is not required to be hemodynamically stable because, being continuous, it allows the slow withdrawal of fluids. And there is also the possibility of correction of metabolic abnormalities by adjusting the concentration of the dialysate.[13,48] The difficulties of continuous methods include, as in the HI, the need for central venous access to allow adequate blood flow, which can be a problem for newborns and small infants. There is also the large volume of extracorporeal circuit (lines and dialyzers) that should not exceed 10% of volemia of the patient (due to the risk of hemodynamic instability), which often forces the system to be primed by filling the circuit with packed red blood cells, besides the technological complexity and the high cost. [48]

Prognosis of the NB with AKI

AKI has been recognized as an independent prognostic factor in critically ill patients and mortality and associated risk factors have been widely studied. [9,16,19,23,24]. For instance, in a study recently published by Askenazi DJ [50], the author observed after the controlling of demographic characteristics, complications, comorbidities and interventions that AKI was an independent risk factor for mortality with an OR of 2. Similar studies in adults and children with AKI showed an increased OR for mortality compared with patients without AKI.[9,20,21,23,24] However, there is little information about long-term prognosis. Recently, clinical, experimental and review studies have drawn attention to the occurrence of impaired renal function, proteinuria and hypertension after episodes of AKI, regardless of the cause of it. Furthermore, cohort studies have shown even in patients with normal creatinine (for age) at discharge, occurrence of renal changes after a few years. Thus, there is a need for monitoring renal function, and for controlling proteinuria and blood pressure levels of these patients. [1,8,10,16,26]

Conclusion

Several efforts have been made in order to improve the assessment of renal function in newborns, to test definitions and classification systems, and also to develop new biomarkers for AKI. Newborns have unique characteristics that defy our ability to understand AKI. Unquestionably, there is a need for multicenter studies to enable us "to find" the best method for the assessment of renal function and for diagnosis of AKI in newborns. So far, studies suggest that critically ill neonates have high rates of AKI with a guarded prognosis. Moreover, newborns with AKI can evolve with impairment of renal function, proteinuria and hypertension requiring long term monitoring. Appropriate evaluation of renal function represents, therefore, the first step towards the recognition and early treatment of AKI (elimination of risk factors) and a change in short and long-term prognosis of critically ill newborns.

References

[1] Cavagnaro F. (2010). Insuficiencia renal aguda en recien nascidos. *Arch. Latin Nefr. Ped*, 10,16-24.

[2] Rodrigues MM, Gomez A, Abitbol C, Chandar J, Montane B, Zilleruelo G.(2005). Comparative renal histomorphometry: a case study of oligonephrophaty of prematurity. *Pediatr Nephrol*, 20,945-949.

[3] Ringer AS. (2010). Acute renal failure in the neonate. NeoReviews,11,e243-e251.

[4] Bresolin NL. (2010). Prognóstico em longo prazo da criança com dano renal agudo. *Arch. Latin Nefr. Ped*,10:12-15.

[5] Andreoli S. (2004). Acute renal failure in the newborn. *Semin Perinatol*, 28,112-123.

[6] Hoste EA, Damen J, Vanholder RC, Lameire NH, Delanghe JR, Van den Hauwe K et al. (2005). Assesment of renal function in recently admitted critically ill patient with normal serum creatinine. *Nephrol Dial Transplant*, 20,747-753.

[7] Armangil D, Yurdakök M, Canpolat FE, Korkmaz A, Yigit S, Tekinalp G. (2008). Determination of reference values for plasma cystatin C and comparison with creatinine in premature infants. *Pediatr Nephrol*, 23,2081-2083.

[8] Askenazi DJ, Ambalavanan N, Goldstein SL. (2009). Acute kidney injury in critically ill newborns: what do we know? What do we need to learn? *Pediatr Nephrol*, 24,265-274.

[9] Bresolin NL, Silva C, Hallal A, Toporovski J, Fernandes V, Goes J, ET al. (2009). Prognosis for children with acute kidney injury in the intensive care unit. *Pediatr Nephrol*, 24:537-544.

[10] Abitbol C, Bauer CR, Montane B, Chandar J, Duara S, Zilleruelo G. (2003). Long-term follow-up of extremely low birth weight infants with neonatal renal failure. *Pediatr Nephrol*,18,887-893.

[11] Barletta GM, Bunchman TE. (2004). Acute renal failure in children and infants. *Curr. Opin. Crit. Care*,10:449-504.

[12] Mogal NE, Emblenton ND. (2006). Management of acute renal failure in the newborn. *Seminars in Fetal and Neonatal Medicine*,11,201-213.

[13] Bresolin NL, Freddi NA. (2002). Insuficiência renal aguda no período neonatal. In: Cruz J, Cruz HMM, Barros RT (Eds), *Atualidades em Nefrologia 7* (PP 386-396). São Paulo: Sarvier.

[14] Nobilis A, Kocsis I, Toth-Heyn P. (2001). Variance of ACE and ATL receptor genotype does not influence the risk of neonatal acute renal failure. *Pediatr Nephrol*, 16, 1063-1066.

[15] Treszl A, Toth-Heyn P, Kocsis I. (2002). Interleukin genetic variants and the risk of renal failure in infants with infecction. *Pediatr Nephrol*,17, 713-717.

[16] Andreoli SP. Acute kidney injury in children. (2009). *Pediatr Nephrol*, 24,253-263.

[17] Suen WS, Mok CK, Chiu SW, Cheung KL, Lee WT, Cheung D, et al. (1998). Risk
      Factors for development of acute renal failure (ARF) requiring dialysis in patient
      undergoing cardiac surgery. *Angiology*, 49(10),789-800.

[18] Huang SC, Wu ET, Chen YS, Chang CI, Chiu IS, Chi NH, et al. (2005). Experience
      with extracorporeal life support in pediatric patients after cardiac surgery. *ASAIO
      Journal*, 51,517:521.

[19] Sheridan AM, Boneventre J. (2000). Cell biology and molecular mechanisms of injury
      in ischemic acute renal failure. *Curr. Opin. Nephrol. Hypertens*, 9,427-429.

[20] Bellomo R, Ronco CF, Kellum JA, Metha RL, Palevski P. (2004). Acute Dialysis
      Quality Initiative Workgroup Acute renal failure – definition, outcomes measures,
      animal modes, fluid therapy and information technology needs. *Crit. Care*, 8,R204-
      R212.

[21] Akcan-Arikan A, Zappitelli M, Loftis LL, Washburn KK, Jefferson LS, Goldstein SL.
      (2007). Modified RIFLE criteria in critically ill children with acute kidney injury.
      Kidney Int, 71,1028-1035.

[22] Duzova A, Bakkalogu A, Kalyoncu M, Poyrazoglu H, Delibas A, Ozkaya O, et al.
      (2010). Etiology and outcome of acute kidney injury in children. *Pediatr Nephrol*,
      25,1453-1461.

[23] Plotz FB, Bouma AB, van Wijk JAE, Kneyber MCJ, Böekenkamp A. (2008). Pediatric
      acute kidney injury in the ICU: an independent evaluation of pRIFLE criteria. *Intensive
      Care Med*, 34,1713-1717.

[24] Freire KMS, Bresolin NL, Farah CF, Carvalho FLC, Góes JEC. (2010). Lesão renal
      aguda em crianças: incidência e fatores prognósticos em crianças gravemente enfermas.
      Rev. Bras. Ter. Intensiva, 22(2),99-102.

[25] Gouyon JB, Guignard JP. (2000). Management of acute renal failure in newborns.
      Pediatr Nephrol,14,1037-1044.

[26] Mak RH. (2008) Acute kidney injury in children: the dawn of a new era. *Pediatr
      Nephrol*, 23,2147-2149.

[27] Pannu N, Nadim MK. (2008). An overview of drug-induced acute kidney injury. *Crit.
      Care Med*, 36[suppl]:S216-223.

[28] Schwartz GJ, Furth SL. (2007). Glomerular filtration rate measurement and estimation
      in chronic kidney disease. *Pediatr Nephrol*, 22,1839-1848.

[29] Vogt BA, Avner ED. (2002). The kidney and urinary tract. In: Fanaroff AA, Martin RJ
      (EDs), *Neonatal Perinatal Medicine Diseases of the fetus and infant*. 7th ed (pp 1517-
      1536). St Louis: Mosby.

[30] Kim MS, Herrin JT. (2008). Renal conditions. In: Cloherty JP, Eichenwald EC, Stark
      AR (eds), Manual of Neonatal Care 6th ed (PP. 587-607). Philadelphia:Wolters Kluwer.

[31] Rudd PT Huges EA, Placzek MM. (1983) Reference ranges for plasma creatinine
      during the first month of life. *Arch. Dis. Child*, 58,212-215.

[32] Van den AnKer JN, de Groot R, Broerse HM. (1995) Assesment of glomerular
      filtration rate in preterm infants by serum creatinine: Comparison with insulin
      clearance. *Pediatrics*, 96, 1156-1158.

[33] Schwartz JG, Brian LP, Spitzer A. (1987). The use of plasma creatinine concentration
      for estimating glomerular filtration rate in infants, children and adolescents. Pediatr
      Clin. North Am, 34, 571-590.

[34] Lameire N, Hoste E. Reflections on the definition, classification, and diagnostic evaluation of acute renal failure. (2004). *Curr. Opin. Crit. Care*,10:468-475.

[35] Lassnigg A, Schmidlin D, Mouhieddine M, Bachmann LM, Druml W, Bauer P et al. (2004). Minimal changes of serum creatinine predict prognosis in patients after cardiothoracic surgery: a prospective cohort study. *J. Am. Soc. Nephrol*, 15,1597-1605.

[36] Daschner M. (2005). Drug dosage in children with reduced renal function. *Pediatr Nephrol*, 20,1675-1686.

[37] Mishra J, Dent C, Tarabish R, Mitsnefes MM, Ma Q, Kelly C et al. Neutrophil gelatinase-associated lipocalin (NGAL) as a biomarker for acute renal injury after cardiac surgery. (2005) *Lancet*, 365,1231-1238.

[38] Devarajan P. (2008). The future of pediatric acute kidney injury management – biomarkers. *Semin. Nephrol*, 28, 493-498.

[39] Zappitelli M. (2008). Epidemiology and diagnosis of acute kidney injury. *Semin. Nephrol*,28,436-446.

[40] Stevens LA, Coresh J, Greene T, Levey AS. (2006). Medical progress assessing kidney function – measured and estimated glomerular filtration rate. *N. Engl. J. Med*, 354, 2473-2483.

[41] Armangil D, Yurdakök M, Canpolat FE, Korkmaz A, Yigit S, Tekinalp G. (2008). Determination of reference values of plasma cystatin C and comparison with creatinine in premature infants. *Pediatr Nephrol*, 23,2081-2083.

[42] Andersen TB, Eskild-Jensen A, Frokiaeer J, Brochner-Mortensen J. (2009) Measuring glomerular filtration rate in children; can cystatin C replace established methods? A review. *Pediatr Nephrol*,24, 929-941.

[43] Bestic M, reed MD. (2005) Common diuretics used in the preterm and term infant. *Neoreviews*, 6,392-398.

[44] Kellum JA, Decker JM. (2001). Use of dopamine in acute renal failure: a meta-analysis. *Crit. Care Med*, 29,1526-1531.

[45] Landoni G, Biondi-Zoccai GG, Tumlin JA, Bove T, De Luca M, Calabró MG et AL. (2007). Beneficial impact of fenoldopam in critically ill patients with or at risk for acute renal feilure: a meta-analysis of randomized clinical trials. *Am. J. Dis*, 49,56-68.

[46] Knoderer CA, Leiser JD, Nailescu C, Turrentine MW, Andreoli SP. (2008). Fenoldopam for acute kidney injury in children. *Pediatr Nephrol*, 23,495-498.

[47] Haycock GB. (2009). Management of acute and chronic renal failure in the newborn. *Seminars in Neonatology*, 8, 325-324.

[48] Walters S, Porter C, Brophy PD. (2009). Dialysis and pediatric acute kidney injury: choice of renal support modality. *Pediatr Nephrol*, 24,37-48.

[49] Akcay A, Turkmen K, Lee DW, Edelstein C. (2010). Update on the diagnosis and mangement of acute kidney injury. *International Journal of Nephrology and Renovascular Disease*, 10,129-140.

[50] Askenazi DJ. (2009). *Acute kidney injury is independently associated with mortality in very low birthweight infants: a matched case-control analysis Pediatr Nephrol*, 24,991-997.

In: Acute Kidney Injury: Causes, Diagnosis and Treatments   ISBN: 978-1-61209-790-9
Editor: Jonathan D. Mendoza, pp. 37-49   © 2011 Nova Science Publishers, Inc.

Chapter III

Kidney Ischemia and Reperfusion Injury

Valquiria Bueno[*]

Head of the Laboratory of Experimental Models in Immunology
UNIFESP Federal University of São Paulo - Immunology Division
São Paulo – Brazil

Abstract

Acute kidney injury (AKI) is an important occurrence characterized by a sudden decrease in renal function. Acute kidney injury (AKI) caused by ischemia and reperfusion injury (IRI) is a common clinical syndrome, associated with high morbidity and mortality. Much of the increased risk of death associated with AKI is from non-renal complications, usually related to multi-organ dysfunction.

Serum creatinine which has been considered the main diagnostic test for AKI rises late in the pathophysiology and is an inaccurate marker of acute changes in glomerular filtration rate. New biomarkers are in evaluation with the aim to identify a possible AKI before oliguria or elevated serum creatinine is detectable, as those criteria already reflect established renal tubular cell injury. Toll-like receptors (TLR), neutrophil gelatinase-associated lipocalin (NGAL), liver-type fatty acid binding protein (L-FABP) or kidney injury molecule-1 (KIM-1) which levels increase prior to the serum creatinine elevation are promising and have been used in clinical trials.

In kidney transplantation the occurrence of ischemia and reperfusion injury (IRI) can delay graft function with the need of postoperative dialysis. Also IRI has been associated with chronic allograft rejection and has influence on long-term graft survival. Our group showed recently that as early as 24 hours after kidney ischemia and reperfusion injury in mice a significant increase of TLR2 and TLR4 expression occurs not only on resident cells but also in kidney infiltrating cells (leukocytes). The increase in these markers was associated with the decrease of kidney function (as depicted by the increase in serum creatinine and urea levels) and acute tubular necrosis. The use of an immunomodulatory agent (FTY720) decreased TLR levels and provided earlier recovery

[*] E-mail: valquiria@nefro.epm.br

of renal function with no effect on kidney structure. These data suggest that studies for the discovery of new biomarkers with early expression and the restriction of inflammatory responses are promising tools for diagnosis and therapies to reduce acute kidney injury.

Kidney Ischemia and Reperfusion Injury

Ischemia-reperfusion injury (IRI) occurs in many clinical situations including myocardial infarction, stroke, trauma, sepsis and transplantation. There are notable quantitative and qualitative differences in ischemia-reperfusion injury response in organs such as kidney, heart, and brain. Acute kidney injury (AKI) caused by IRI is a common clinical syndrome, associated with high morbidity and mortality [1, 2]. Much of the increased risk of death associated with AKI is from non-renal complications [3], usually related to multi-organ dysfunction.

Cessation of arterial blood flow with immediate oxygen deprivation in cells (i.e., hypoxia with accumulation of metabolic products) is defined as ischemic injury. In the kidney, decreased blood supply is associated with flow diversion from cortex to medulla which preserves oxygenation of the metabolically vulnerable medulla at the expense of cortical perfusion and glomerular filtration [4]. Sensitivity to hypoxia or ischemia has been demonstrated in both proximal tubules [5] and their thick ascending limbs [6].

Severe reduction of renal blood flow causes cell damage both by the high-energy phosphate depletion and the subsequent failure to maintain physiological ion gradients across the cell membrane. However, the major injury to the ischemic organ occurs during the reperfusion phase in which the blood flow returns to the ischemic tissue. Reperfusion is associated with free radical generation leading to lipid peroxidation, polysaccharide depolymerization and deoxyribonucleotide degradation. Injured endothelial cells fail to vasodilate underlying vascular smooth muscle, release potent vasoconstrictors and swell which leads to increased permeability [4].

In addition IRI induces inflammatory responses as it follows:

- Oxygen deprivation due to ischemia induces early ATP depletion which stops ATP-dependent transport pumps, resulting in mitochondrial swelling. Mitochondrial swelling results in outer membrane rupture, with release of mitochondrial intermembrane proteins. Caspase 1 or interleukin-1 converting enzyme (ICE) cleaves interleukin (IL)-1b. IL-1b is a pro-inflammatory cytokine, and can induce renal tubular epithelial cells to secrete chemokines such as keratinocyte-induced chemoattractant (KC), macrophage inflammatory protein (MIP)-1a, or RANTES [7].
- Hypoxia inducible factor (HIF-1, HIF-2, HIF-3), HIF-3 may be a negative regulator of hypoxia-inducible genes expressed by HIF-1 and HIF-2 [8]. HIF-1 is unstable under normal conditions but is stable and works under hypoxic conditions [9, 10]. Many genes encoding for cytokines and growth factors are induced by HIF-1 activation [11, 12].
- Oxygen-derived free radicals, in particular hydrogen peroxide, which is a source of oxygen-derived free radicals after IRI injury, has been reported to induce TNF-α production by activating p38 mitogen-activated protein kinase (MAPK) [13].

Following kidney IRI, the coordinated action of cytokines/chemokines, reactive oxygen intermediates and adhesion molecules causes a cascade of events leading to endothelial cell dysfunction, tubular epithelial cell injury and activation of both tissue-resident and kidney infiltrating leukocytes [14, 15].

Vascular Endothelial Cells

Activation of the endothelium following kidney IRI leads to a loss of vascular endothelial cell integrity [16, 17] and up-regulation of adhesion molecules such as intracellular adhesion molecule 1 (ICAM-1) and P-selectin [18, 19, 20] thus facilitating leukocyte-endothelial cell interactions. Also, endothelial cells from the injured kidney produce chemokines which mediate the recruitment of macrophages expressing CX_3CR1 and CCR2 to this inflammatory site [21, 22]. Therefore, the endothelium, which serves as the interface between immune cells and the renal parenchyma is a highly reactive tissue involved in the early phase of inflammation and kidney damage by promoting the accumulation of leukocytes.

Tubular Epithelial Cells

The basolateral membrane of proximal tubule cells expresses the complement inhibitor, Crry. After renal IRI, Crry is internalized allowing the deposition of complement component 3 (C3) on the tubular epithelium [23], complement activation and production of the pro-inflammatory chemokines macrophage inflammatory factor-2 (MIP-2) and keratinocyte-derived chemokine (KC) [24]. These chemokines attract neutrophils and macrophages to the post-ischemic kidney. In addition, toll-like receptors (TLR) 2 and 4 are up-regulated in epithelial cells after IR.

Activation of Kidney Resident Cells and Kidney-Infiltrating Leukocytes

Dendritic Cells (DCs - CD11c$^+$) and class II major histocompatibility complex (MHC Class II)$^+$ DCs are the most abundant leukocyte subset residing in the normal mouse kidney [22, 25] suggesting an important role in renal immunity and inflammation. TNF-α, IL-6, MCP-1 and RANTES (pro-inflammatory cytokines/chemokines) are produced by renal DCs after IRI, and depletion of DCs prior to IRI significantly reduced the kidney levels of TNF-α [26].

Neutrophils inhibition has been shown in some studies to attenuate renal injury after IRI [27], whereas other studies failed to find a protective effect of neutrophil blockade or depletion [28]. Many factors affecting neutrophil infiltration or activation including neutrophil elastase, tissue-type plasminogen activator, hepatocyte growth factor, and CD44 have been suggested to contribute for the renal injury following IRI [29, 30, 31, 32]. Despite discrepancies in data provided by different research groups, it is likely that neutrophils participate in inducing renal injury by plugging renal microvasculature and releasing oxygen-free radicals and proteases.

Macrophages infiltrate the injured kidney early within 1 hour of reperfusion, and this infiltration is mediated by CCR2 [22] and CX_3CR1 signaling pathways [21, 22]. Analysis of kidney infiltrating macrophages by flow cytometry demonstrated that these leukocytes are significant producers of the cytokines IL-1α, IL-6, IL-12p40/70 and TNF-α [22].

Natural Killer (NK) cells have recently been reported to infiltrate the post-ischemic kidney by 4 hours of reperfusion. IRI induced the expression of an NK cell-activating ligand (Rae-1) on tubule epithelial cells (TECs) and *in vitro* studies demonstrated that the interaction of the NKG2D receptor on NK cells with Rae-1 on TECs causes perforin-dependent lysis of cultured kidney cells. Antibody-mediated depletion of NK cells inhibited IRI in wild-type (WT) mice and adoptive transfer of NK cells from WT, but not from perforin KO mice into T, B and NK cell-deficient mice enhanced IRI [33].

Invariant Natural Killer T (iNKT) cells are a unique subset of T lymphocytes with surface receptors and functional properties shared with conventional T cells and NK cells. In contrast to conventional T cells, iNKT cells are activated by endogenously released glycolipid antigens. A recent finding is that the number of IFN-γ producing iNKT cells in the kidney is significantly increased by 3 hours of reperfusion compared to sham-operated mice. Also, blockade of NKT cell activation with the anti-CD1d mAb, NKT cell depletion with an anti-NK1.1 mAb in WT mice, or use of iNKT cell deficient mice ($Jα18^{-/-}$) inhibited the accumulation of IFN-γ producing neutrophils after IRI and prevented AKI [34].

T Lymphocytes

In the early stage of IRI, T cells may become activated through antigen-independent mechanisms by inflammatory cytokines and reactive oxygen intermediates [35]. T cell trafficking was observed as early as 1 h after IRI and decreased at 24 h following IRI [36, 37]. T cell recruitment influences proinflammatory cytokine production, neutrophil trafficking, and progression to fibrosis [38].

Moreover, T cells also influence vascular permeability in early ischemic AKI [39]. Increased numbers of activated and effector-memory T cells were found in the postischemic kidneys as late as 6 weeks after IRI, suggesting that T cells are also involved in long term structural changes of postischemic kidneys [40].

Increased Factors after IRI

Adhesion Molecules

IRI causes cytokine synthesis, altered cell adhesion, leukocyte migration and leukocyte-mediated tissue damage [41]. Cell migration is mediated by the increase of leukocyte adhesion molecules such as CD11/CD18 (β2 integrin), intercellular adhesion molecule-1 (ICAM-1) and selectins which have been used as targets to attenuate IRI in experimental models [42, 43, 44].

Cytokines and Chemokines

IRI stimulates the synthesis of pro-inflammatory cytokines including IL-1, IL-6, and TNF-α [45]. The blockade of IL-1, IL-6, and keratinocyte-derived chemokine (KC; a mouse analog of human IL-8) reduces renal injury in murine renal IRI models [46]. Chemokines also play a role in the pathogenesis of renal injury in the postischemic kidneys. The synthesis of growth-related oncogene (GRO)-α/KC increased in the postischemic kidneys in a murine renal IRI model [47] and the neutralization of GRO-α/KC and macrophage inflammatory protein-2 mitigated renal injury [48]. CXCR3 expression is induced in the postischemic kidneys and CXCR3-deficient mice are protected from renal injury after IRI [49].

Blockade of CX3CR1 reduced inflammation and interstitial fibrosis in the postischemic kidneys, suggesting that a blockade of CX3CR1 signaling pathway may contribute to protect kidneys from IRI [50].

Fractalkine (CX3CL1), which is expressed on injured endothelial cells, is a potent chemoattractant and adhesion molecule for macrophages carrying the fractalkine receptor (CX3CR1). CX3CL1 expression is increased on vascular endothelium of postischemic kidneys and CX3CR1 inhibition by a specific antibody resulted in reduced macrophage infiltration and partial kidney protection [21].

Hypoxia-Inducible Factor

Activation of hypoxia-inducible factor (HIF) occurs in tubular, interstitial, and endothelial cells after IRI. HIF-1 was reported to affect infiltration of macrophages in postischemic kidneys [51] and cobalt which inhibits HIF-1 degradation, protected rats from renal injury by reducing macrophage infiltration into the kidneys after IRI [52].

Carbon monoxide or HIF prolyl hydroxylases inhibitors significantly reduced serum creatinine at 24 and 72 h after IRI and attenuated renal tubular injury at 72 h in rats, suggesting that inhibited activation of HIF may improve both short- and long-term outcomes after IRI [53].

Toll-Like Receptors

Toll-like receptors (TLRs) are a family of transmembrane proteins that in addition of binding to a range of microbial products can also recognize endogenous ligands termed danger-associated molecular patterns (DAMPs). TLR2 and TLR4 bind to heat shock proteins, high mobility group box 1 (HMGB1), breakdown products of fibronectin, heparan sulfate, and hyaluronic acid. TLR2 and TLR4 are constitutively expressed in both proximal and distal tubules, the thin limb of the loop of Henle and the collecting ducts with upregulation in these areas after IRI [54].

On activation of the TLR occurs an intracellular cascade of events resulting in the release of NF-κB from IκB, allowing NF-κB to translocate from cytoplasm to the nucleus and mediate an increase in inflammatory cytokine gene expression which leads to pro-inflammatory responses [55, 56].

Changes in Renal Tissue after IRI

During ischemic injury, subsets of proximal tubular cells (most susceptible to this injury) detach from the extracellular matrix (ECM) due to cellular junctional complexes breakdown [57, 58, 59], lose plasma membrane polarity [60, 61] and are expelled into the tubule lumen and observed as cell casts in the urine. Cellular debris can form tubular obstructions and all these processes contribute to pathophysiological consequences of ischemia.

Ischemia results in disruption and dysregulation of the actin cytoskeleton, and loss of cell-cell and cell-ECM attachments. Following severe injury, cells can become dedifferentiated, taking on characteristics of early development such as loss of surface membrane polarity. Regaining the polarized phenotype involves participation of both integrins and CAMs (cellular adhesion molecules). With very severe injury, cells can die either via cell necrosis (rare) or apoptosis [62].

Bcl-2 (pro-apoptotic and anti-apoptotic family of genes) polypeptides localize into intracellular sites where reactive oxygen species are generated and they have been shown to inhibit apoptosis via an anti-oxidant pathway that prevents cellular damage by reactive oxygen species [63]. The balance between anti-apoptotic and pro-apoptotic increased genes expression play a role in the regeneration and repair following IRI.

During the early phase after IRI the findings in renal tissue are necrosis of tubule cells and infiltration of inflammatory cells. Tubular epithelial cells may produce growth factors including FGF, TGF-a, EGF-like growth factor, IL-2, and osteopontin at regenerative wound margins associated with leukocyte infiltration [64, 65, 66] leading to necrotic area repair and renal function recovery. Furuichi et al. suggested that inhibitory mechanisms to control excessive cell proliferation also play a role and they found that IP-10 had an inhibitory effect on tubular cell proliferation *in vivo* and *in vitro*. The interstitial infiltrated F4/80-positive cells were the main source of IP-10 [67]. Other cells including bone marrow derived stem cells or intra-renal mesenchymal stem cells might participate in the kidney regeneration [68].

However, if the IRI is too damaging or not appropriately treated, chronic kidney disease occurs. Chronic fibrotic changes are characterized by an expansion of the interstitial area, leukocyte infiltration and the production of extracellular matrix [69, 70]. Kim et al. [71] showed that reactive oxygen species (ROS) induces interstitial cell proliferation with subsequent renal insufficiency via the expansion of the interstitial area and extracellular matrix deposition. Moreover, ROS inhibited the proliferation of tubular epithelial cells required for the restoration of renal function after IRI. When mice submitted to IRI were treated earlier and for a long period with a cell permeable superoxide dismutase (SOD) mimetic MnTMPyP, there was a dramatic attenuation in the interstitial myofibroblasts proliferation suggesting that ROS is a critical factor in the induction of fibrotic changes in post ischemic kidneys.

In addition to fibroblast leading to chronic kidney disease, fibrocytes which are circulating connective tissue cell progenitors have shown to play a role in this process [72]. Kidney-infiltrating inflammatory cells produce transforming growth factor (TGF)-b and platelet-derived growth factor (PDGF) which are fibrosis-promoting factors [73]. Also, CX3CL1/fractalkine and its unique receptor CX3CR1 are upregulated after IRI and participate in the pathogenesis of renal fibrosis. They cause the accumulation of macrophages and platelets in the outer medulla with the expression of macrophage and platelet-derived fibrogenic protein platelet-derived growth factor-B [50].

FTY720 Modulates the Inflammatory Process after IRI (74)

We evaluated the effects of IRI at early time point (24 hours) in C57BL/6 mice submitted to 30 minutes of bilateral renal pedicle clamp and treated with FTY720 (single i.v. dose 1mg/kg). FTY720-treated (IR+FTY) mice presented a significant decrease at serum levels of creatinine and urea in comparison with non-treated mice (IR) submitted to IRI as shown in Figure 1. However, acute tubular necrosis was similar when groups were compared.

We also observed that spleen cells from treated mice presented a significant lower expression of TLR2 and TLR4 when compared with non-treated mice. These data suggest that FTY720 prevents inflammatory cells activation mainly by inhibiting TLR activation (Figure 2).

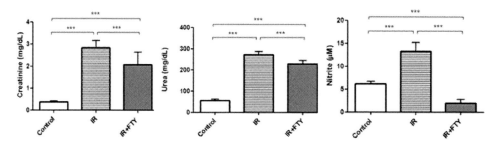

Figure 1. Serum creatinine (A), serum urea (B) and serum nitrite (C) in control mice, 24 hours after ischemia/reperfusion injury non-treated (IR) and FTY720-treated mice (IR+FTY). *** p<0,0001.

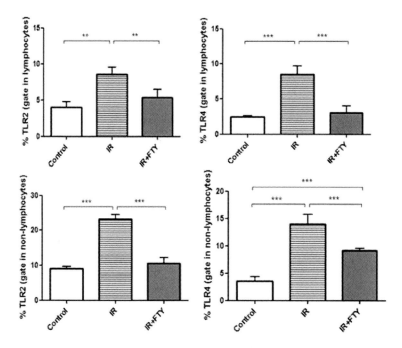

Figure 2. Percentage of spleen lymphocytes TLR2[+] (A), spleen non-lymphocytes TLR2[+] (B), spleen lymphocytes TLR4[+] (C) and spleen non-lymphocytes TLR4[+] (D) in control mice, 24 hours after ischemia/reperfusion injury non-treated (IR) and FTY720-treated mice (IR+FTY). **p=0,001; ***p<0,0001.

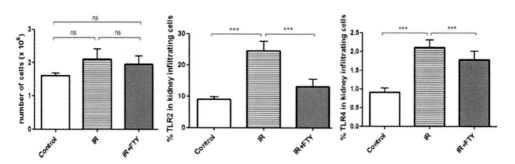

Figure 3. Number of kidney infiltrating cells (KIC) (A), percentage of KIC TLR2$^+$ (B), and percentage of KIC TLR4$^+$ (C) in control mice, 24 hours after ischemia/reperfusion injury non-treated (IR) and FTY720-treated mice (IR+FTY). Ns=not significant (p=0,069); ***p<0,0001.

The same was observed (Figure 3) for the kidney infiltrating cells (KIC) suggesting that FTY720 modulates the activation of the immune response after IRI not only at periphery but also at the inflammatory site (kidney).

When IL-6/actin ratio was measured in the renal tissue by Western blot, we found an increased level in non-treated group (IR) when compared with control mice (IR=41.8±3.5 versus Control= 6.8±0.08). FTY720 treatment decreased the levels of the pro-inflammatory cytokine IL-6 in the renal tissue (IR+FTY=15.0±1.3).

In conclusion, several events are associated with kidney damage after IRI and as shown by our data and confirmed by others the modulation of the inflammatory response seems crucial to provide early kidney recovery.

References

[1]   Star RA. Treatment of acute renal failure. *Kidney International* 1998; 54: 1817–1831.

[2]   Palevsky PM, Zhang JH, O'Connor TZ, Chertow GM, Crowley ST, Choudhury D, et al. Intensity of renal support in critically ill patients with acute kidney injury. *New England Journal of Medic*ine 2008; 359: 7–20.

[3]   Chertow GM, Levy EM, Hammermeister KE, Grover F, Daley J. Independent association between acute renal failure and mortality following cardiac surgery. *American Journal of Medicine* 1998; 104:343–348.

[4]   Woolfson RG, Millar CGM, Neild GH. Ischaemia and reperfusion injury in the kidney: current status and future direction. *Nephrology Dialysis and Transplantation* 1994; 9(11): 1529-1531.

[5]   Shanley P, Brezis M, Spokes K, Silva P, Epstein F, Rosen S. Hypoxic injury in the proximal tubule of the isolated perfused rat kidney. *Kidney International* 1986; 29: 1021-1032.

[6]   Brezis M, Shanley P, Silva P et al. Disparate mechanisms for hypoxic injury in different nephron segments. Studies in the isolated perfused rat kidney. *Journal of Clinical Investigation* 1985; 76: 1796-1806.

[7]   Furuichi K, Wada T, Iwata Y, Sakai N, Yoshimoto K, Kobayashi Ki K, et al. Administration of FR167653, a new anti-inflammatory compound, prevents renal

ischaemia/reperfusion injury in mice. *Nephrology Dialysis and Transplantation* 2002; 17: 399–407.

[8] Nangaku M, Inagi R, Miyata T, Fujita T. Hypoxia and hypoxia inducible factor in renal disease. *Nephron Experimental Nephrology* 2008; 110: e1–7.

[9] Huang LE, Arany Z, Livingston DM, Bunn HF. Activation of hypoxia-inducible transcription factor depends primarily upon redox-sensitive stabilization of its alpha subunit. *The Journal of Biological Chemistry* 1996; 271: 32253–32259.

[10] Salceda S, Caro J. Hypoxia-inducible factor 1alpha (HIF-1alpha) protein is rapidly degraded by the ubiquitin-proteasome system under normoxic conditions. Its stabilization by hypoxia depends on redox-induced changes. *The Journal of Biological Chemistry* 1997; 272: 22642–22647.

[11] El Awad B, Kreft B, Wolber EM, Hellwig-Burgel T, Metzen E, Fandrey J, et al. Hypoxia and interleukin-1beta stimulate vascular endothelial growth factor production in human proximal tubular cells. *Kidney International* 2000; 58: 43–50.

[12] Zhou J, Brune B. Cytokines and hormones in the regulation of hypoxia inducible factor-1alpha (HIF-1alpha). *Cardiovascular and Hematological Agents in Medicinal Chemistry* 2006; 4:189–197.

[13] Meldrum DR, Dinarello CA, Cleveland JC Jr, Cain BS, Shames BD, Meng X, et al. Hydrogen peroxide induces tumor necrosis factor alpha-mediated cardiac injury by a P38 mitogen-activated protein kinase-dependent mechanism. *Surgery* 1998; 124:291–296.

[14] Bonventre JV, Weinberg JM. Recent advances in the pathophysiology of ischemic acute renal failure. *The Journal of American Society of Nephrology* 2003; 14: 2199–2210.

[15] Li L, Okusa MD. Blocking the Immune response in ischemic acute kidney injury: the role of adenosine 2A agonists. *Nature Clinical Practice Nephrology* 2006; 2: 432–444.

[16] Sutton TA, Mang HE, Campos SB, Sandoval RM, Yoder MC, Molitoris BA. Injury of the renal microvascular endothelium alters barrier function after ischemia. *The American Journal of Physiology Renal Physiology* 2003; 285: F191–198.

[17] Brodsky SV, Yamamoto T, Tada T, Kim B, Chen J, Kajiya F, et al. Endothelial dysfunction in ischemic acute renal failure: rescue by transplanted endothelial cells. *The American Journal of Physiology Renal Physiology* 2002; 282: F1140–1149.

[18] Kelly KJ, Williams WW, Colvin RB, Meehan SM, Springer TA, Gutierrez-Ramos J, et al. Intercellular adhesion molecule-1-deficient mice are protected against ischemic renal injury. *Journal of Clinical Investigation* 1996; 97: 1056–1063.

[19] Singbartl K, Green SA, Ley K. Blocking P-selectin protects from ischemia/reperfusion-induced acute renal failure. *The FASEB Journal* 2000; 14: 48–54.

[20] Okusa MD, Linden J, Huang L, Rieger JM, Macdonald TL, Huynh LP. A2a-Adenosine receptor mediated inhibition of renal injury and neutrophil adhesion. *American Journal of Physiology* 2000; 279: F809–818.

[21] Oh DJ, Dursun B, He Z, Lu L, Hoke TS, Ljubanovic D, et al. Fractalkine receptor (CX3CR1) inhibition is protective against ischemic acute renal failure in mice. *The American Journal of Physiology Renal Physiology* 2008; 294: F264–271.

[22] Li L, Huang L, Sung SS, Vergis AL, Rosin DL, Rose CE, Jr, et al. The chemokine receptors CCR2 and CX3CR1 mediate monocyte/macrophage trafficking in kidney ischemia-reperfusion injury. *Kidney International* 2008; 74: 1526–1537.

[23] Thurman JM, Ljubanovic D, Royer PA, Kraus DM, Molina H, Barry NP, et al. Altered renal tubular expression of the complement inhibitor Crry permits complement activation after ischemia/reperfusion. *The Journal of Clinical Investigation* 2006; 116: 357–368.

[24] Thurman JM, Lenderink AM, Royer PA, Coleman KE, Zhou J, Lambris JD, et al. C3a is required for the production of CXC chemokines by tubular epithelial cells after renal ischemia/reperfusion. *The Journal of Immunology* 2007; 178: 1819–1828.

[25] Soos TJ, Sims TN, Barisoni L, Lin K, Littman DR, Dustin ML, et al. CX3CR1+ interstitial dendritic cells form a contiguous network throughout the entire kidney. *Kidney International* 2006; 70: 591–596.

[26] Dong X, Swaminathan S, Bachman LA, Croatt AJ, Nath KA, Griffin MD. Resident dendritic cells are the predominant TNF-secreting cell in early renal ischemia-reperfusion injury. *Kidney Int.* 2007; 71:619–28.

[27] Kelly KJ, Williams WW Jr, Colvin RB et al. (1996) Intercellular adhesion molecule-1-deficient mice are protected against ischemic renal injury. *Journal of Clinical Investigation* 1996; 97:1056–1063.

[28] Thornton MA, Winn R, Alpers CE, Zager RA. An evaluation of the neutrophil as a mediator of in vivo renal ischemic–reperfusion injury. *American Journal of Pathology* 1989; 135:509–515.

[29] Hayama T, Matsuyama M, Funao K et al. Beneficial effect of neutrophil elastase inhibitor on renal warm ischemia– reperfusion injury in the rat. *Transplantation Proceedings* 2006; 38:2201–2202.

[30] Roelofs JJ, Rouschop KM, Leemans JC et al. Tissue-type plasminogen activator modulates inflammatory responses and renal function in ischemia reperfusion injury. *The Journal of American Society of Nephrology* 2006;17:131–140.

[31] Mizuno S, Nakamura T. Prevention of neutrophil extravasation by hepatocyte growth factor leads to attenuations of tubular apoptosis and renal dysfunction in mouse ischemic kidneys. *American Journal of Pathology* 2005; 166:1895–1905.

[32] Rouschop KM, Roelofs JJ, Claessen N et al. Protection against renal ischemia reperfusion injury by CD44 disruption. *The Journal of American Society of Nephrology* 2005; 16:2034–2043.

[33] Zhang ZX, Wang S, Huang X, Min WP, Sun H, Liu W, et al. NK cells induce apoptosis in tubular epithelial cells and contribute to renal ischemia-reperfusion injury. *The Journal of Immunology* 2008; 181:7489–7498.

[34] Li L, Huang L, Sung SJ, Lobo PI, Brown MG, Gregg RK, et al. NKT cell activation mediates neutrophil IFN-gamma production and renal ischemia-reperfusion injury. *The Journal of Immunology* 2007; 178:5899–5911.

[35] Bacon KB, Premack BA, Gardner P, Schall TJ. Activation of dual T cell signaling pathways by the chemokine RANTES. *Science* 1995; 269:1727–1730.

[36] Noiri E, Doi K, Inagi R, Nangaku M, Fujita T. Contribution of T lymphocytes to rat renal ischemia/reperfusion injury. *Clinical Experimental Nephrology* 2009; 13:25–32.

[37] Ascon DB, Lopez-Briones S, Liu M, Ascon M, Savransky V, Colvin RB, et al. Phenotypic and functional characterization of kidney-infiltrating lymphocytes in renal ischemia reperfusion injury. *The Journal of Immunology*; 2006; 177:3380–3387.

[38] Burne MJ, Daniels F, El Ghandour A, Mauiyyedi S, Colvin RB, O'Donnell MP, et al. Identification of the CD4 T cell as a major pathogenic factor in ischemic acute renal failure. *Journal of Clinical Investigation* 2001; 108:1283–1290.

[39] Saito H, Kitamoto M, Kato K, Liu N, Kitamura H, Uemura K, et al. Tissue factor and factor V involvement in rat peritoneal fibrosis. *Peritoneal Dialysis International* 2009; 29:340–351.

[40] Ascon M, Ascon DB, Liu M et al. Renal ischemia–reperfusion leads to long term infiltration of activated and effector-memory T lymphocytes. *Kidney International* 2008; 75:526–535.

[41] Rabb H, Star R. Inflammatory response and its consequences in acute renal failure. In: Molitoris B, Finn W, editors. *Acute renal failure: a companion to Brenner and Rector's 'the Kidney'*. Philadelphia: WB Saunders; 2001. p. 89–100.

[42] Rabb H, Mendiola CC, Dietz J, Saba SR, Issekutz TB, Abanilla F, et al. Role of CD11a and CD11b in ischemic acute renal failure in rats. *American Journal of Physiology* 1994; 267:F1052–1058.

[43] Rabb H, Mendiola CC, Saba SR, Dietz JR, Smith CW, Bonventre JV, et al. Antibodies to ICAM-1 protect kidneys in severe ischemic reperfusion injury. *Biochemical and Biophysical Research Communications* 1995; 211: 67–73

[44] Rabb H, Ramirez G, Saba SR, Reynolds D, Xu J, Flavell R, et al. Renal ischemic-reperfusion injury in L-selectin-deficient mice. *American Journal of Physiology* 1996; 271: F408–413.

[45] Donnahoo KK, Meng X, Ayala A, Cain MP, Harken AH, Meldrum DR. Early kidney TNF-alpha expression mediates neutrophil infiltration and injury after renal ischemia–reperfusion. *American Journal of Physiology* 1999; 277:R922–R929.

[46] HaqM, Norman J, Saba SR, Ramirez G, Rabb H. Role of IL-1 in renal ischemic reperfusion injury. *The Journal of American Society of Nephrology* 1998; 9:614–619.

[47] Daemen MA, de Vries B, van't Veer C, Wolfs TG, Buurman WA. Apoptosis and chemokine induction after renal ischemia–reperfusion. *Transplantation* 2001; 71:1007–1011.

[48] Miura M, Fu X, Zhang QW, Remick DG, Fairchild RL. Neutralization of Gro alpha and macrophage inflammatory protein-2 attenuates renal ischemia/reperfusion injury. *American Journal of Pathology* 2001; 159:2137–2145.

[49] Fiorina P, Ansari MJ, Jurewicz M et al. Role of CXC chemokine receptor 3 pathway in renal ischemic injury. *The Journal of American Society of Nephrology* 2006; 17:716–723.

[50] Furuichi K, Gao JL, Murphy PM. Chemokine receptor CX3CR1 regulates renal interstitial fibrosis after ischemia–reperfusion injury. *American Journal of Pathology* 2006; 169:372–387.

[51] Rosenberger C, Griethe W, Gruber G et al. Cellular responses to hypoxia after renal segmental infarction. *Kidney International* 2003; 64:874–886.

[52] Matsumoto M, Makino Y, Tanaka T et al. Induction of renoprotective gene expression by cobalt ameliorates ischemic injury of the kidney in rats. *The Journal of American Society of Nephrology* 2003; 14:1825–1832.

[53] Bernhardt WM, Campean V, Kany S et al. (2006) Preconditional activation of hypoxia-inducible factors ameliorates ischemic acute renal failure. *The Journal of American Society of Nephrology* 2006; 17:1970–1978.

[54] Wolfs TGAM, Buurman WA, Van Schadewijk A, et al. In vivo expression of Toll-like receptor 2 and 4 by renal epithelial cells: IFN-γ and TNF-α mediated up-regulation during inflammation. *The Journal of Immunology* 2002; 168(3):1286–1293.

[55] Liew FY, Xu D, Brint EK, O'Neill LAJ. Negative regulation of Toll-like receptor-mediated immune responses. *Nature Reviews Immunology* 2005; 5(6):446–458.

[56] O'Neill LAJ. How Toll-like receptors signal: what we know and what we don't know. *Current Opinion in Immunology* 2006;18(1):3–9.

[57] Molitoris BA, Falk SA, Dahl RH. Ischemic-induced loss of epithelial polarity. Role of the tight junction. *Journal of Clinical Investigation* 1989; 84: 1334–1339.

[58] Mandel LJ, Bacallao R, Zampighi G. Uncoupling of the molecular "fence" and paracellular "gate" functions in epithelial tight junctions. *Nature* 1993; 361: 552–555.

[59] Kwon O, Nelson J, Sibley RK, et al. Backleak, tight junctions and cell-cell adhesion in postischemic injury to the renal allograft. *Journal of the American Society of Nephrology* 1996; 7: A2907. Abstract.

[60] Molitoris BA, Chan LK, Shapiro JI, et al. Loss of epithelial polarity: a novel hypothesis for reduced proximal tubule Na1 transport following ischemic injury. *Journal of Membrana Biology* 1989; 107: 119–127.

[61] Fish EM, Molitoris BA. Alterations in epithelial polarity and the pathogenesis of disease states. *New England Journal of Medicine* 1994; 330: 1580–1588.

[62] Sutton TA, Molitoris BA. Mechanisms of cellular injury in ischemic ARF. *Semminars in Nephrology* 1998; 18: 490–497.

[63] Hockenbery D, Oltvai Z, Yin X-M, Milliman C, Korsmeyer S. Bcl-2 functions in an antioxidant pathway to prevent apoptosis. *Cell* 1993; 75: 241–251.

[64] Ghielli M, Verstrepen W, Nouwen E, De Broe ME. Regeneration processes in the kidney after acute injury: role of infiltrating cells. *Experimental Nephrology* 1998; 6: 502–507.

[65] Naor D, Sionov RV, Ish-Shalom D. CD44: structure, function, and association with the malignant process. *Advances in Cancer Research* 1997; 71: 241–319.

[66] Lewington AJ, Padanilam BJ, Martin DR, Hammerman MR. Expression of CD44 in kidney after acute ischemic injury in rats. American Journal of Physiology – Regulatory, *Integrative Comparative Physiology* 2000; 278:R247–254.

[67] Furuichi K, Wada T, Kitajikma S, Toyama T, Okumura T, Hara A, et al. IFN-inducible protein 10 (CXCL10) regulates tubular cell proliferation in renal ischemia–reperfusion injury. *Nephron Experimental Nephrology* 2008; 109: c29–38.

[68] Bussolati B, Tetta C, Camussi G. Contribution of stem cells to kidney repair. *American Journal of Nephrology* 2008; 28:813–822.

[69] Basile DP, Donohoe D, Roethe K, Osborn JL. Renal ischemic injury results in permanent damage to peritubular capillaries and influences long-term function. *American Journal of Physiology Renal Physiology* 2001; 281: F887–F899.

[70] Sharma VK, Bologa RM, Xu GP, Li B, Mouradian J, Wang J, Serur D, Rao V, Suthanthiran M. Intragraft TGF-beta 1 mRNA: a correlate of interstitial fibrosis and chronic allograft nephropathy. *Kidney International* 1996; 49: 1297–1303.

[71] Kim J, Jung KJ, Park KM Park. Reactive oxygen species differently regulate renal tubular epithelial and interstitial cell proliferation after ischemia and reperfusion injury. *American Journal of Physiology Renal Physiology* 2010; 298: F1118–F1129.

[72] Wada T, Sakai N, Matsushima K, Kaneko S. Fibrocytes: a new insight into kidney fibrosis. *Kidney International* 2007; 72: 269–273.

[73] Hirschberg R, Wang S. Proteinuria and growth factors in the development of tubulointerstitial injury and scarring in kidney disease. *Current Opinion in Nephrology and Hypertension* 2005; 14: 43–52.

[74] Pedregosa JF, Gomes GN, Franco M, Bueno V. Decrease of TLR2 and TLR4 is associated with less impairment of renal function after IR. *International Immunology* 2010, 22: iii-176.

In: Acute Kidney Injury: Causes, Diagnosis and Treatments   ISBN: 978-1-61209-790-9
Editor: Jonathan D. Mendoza pp. 51-67   © 2011 Nova Science Publishers, Inc.

Chapter IV

Long-Term Prognostic Implication of Post-Angiographic Acute Kidney Injury and Hemodynamic Instability

Tomonori Kimura[1], Yoshitaka Isaka[1] and Terumasa Hayashi[2]
[1]Department of Geriatirc Medicine and Nephrology, Osaka University Graduate School of Medicine, 2-2 Yamadaoka, Suita, Osaka, Japan 585-0871
[2]Department of Nephrology, Rinku General Medical Center, Izumisano Municipal Hospital, 2-23, Rinku-Orai Kita, Izumisano, Osaka, Japan 598-8577

Abstract

Several studies have found that post-angiographic acute kidney injury (AKI) is a risk of long-term mortality after coronary angiography. These studies have also found that acute hemodynamic disturbances requiring hemodynamic support have a strong impact both on the incidence of AKI and on the prognosis after coronary angiography.

The impact of AKI on prognosis might have been affected by hemodynamic factors in these studies because hemodynamic instability in itself is, not only closely related to the incidence of post-angiographic AKI, but also a strong risk factor for the prognosis. Therefore, we aimed to study the impact of AKI on long-term prognosis after coronary angiography among hospital survivors in relation with hemodynamic variables.

We found that AKI is a predictor of long-term prognosis in the whole studied population, however, its impact was attenuated among hemodynamically stable patients. This result suggested that the impact of AKI for the hemodynamically stable patients was attenuated from the overall patients.

As seen in this study, the cause of AKI in itself could affect the long-term prognosis after AKI. In order to evaluate the long-term prognosis of AKI patients, clinicians need to take the cause of AKI into consideration.

Introduction

It goes without saying that acute kidney injury (AKI) has been one of the most important subjects in clinical and basic studies, and the number of clinical studies of AKI is increasing, especially after the recent consensus of AKI [1, 2]. AKI is also known with its wide variety of etiologies, ranging from outpatients to critically ill patients, and risk factors, pre-renal, renal, and post-renal. Clinical studies have demonstrated that AKI is associated not only with the short-term prognosis, but also with long-term prognosis [3-11]. On the other hand, the causes of AKI in themselves, such as sepsis and shock, have strong impact both on the incidence of AKI and on the prognosis after AKI. Clinical studies have often selected the cause of AKI as risk factors for both AKI and prognosis. This fact indicates that the prognosis after AKI might have been affected by the insult of AKI in itself. We wonder whether AKI in itself affects prognosis or whether the insult of AKI affects through AKI (Figure 1) [12]. Therefore, the relationship between AKI and the cause of AKI on the prognosis is confusing and still unclear. We would like to present how we should consider this confusing relationship of cause and outcome in the field of post-angiographic AKI[12]. In this chapter, we would like to describe the prognosis after post-angiographic AKI, while clarifying the etiology of post-angiographic AKI. First, we are going to mention the relationship of post-angiographic AKI and its causes, including hemodynamics. Then we demonstrate the present data, including ours, to consider the impact of AKI and hemodynamics on the prognosis. And finally, we will present our speculation about how to interpret AKI in the clinical setting and give a future perspective.

Post-Angiograhic AKI

Post-angiograhic AKI is a clinically important problem. This AKI form accounts for one of the most common cause of AKI in hospitalized patients [13, 14]. The term, contrast-induced nephropathy (CIN), or contrast-induced AKI (CIAKI), has been used to express AKI occurring after the usage of contrast media in the angiographic procedure (Figure 2). The usage of contrast medium in itself during the procedure has been regarded as the cause of this type of AKI.

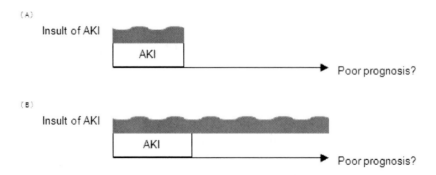

Figure 1. The relationship between AKI, insult of AKI, and prognosis. At the moment, it seems uncertain whether AKI in itself affects prognosis (A) or whether the insult of AKI affects through AKI (B).

> ✓ CIN (contrast-induced nephropathy)
> ✓ CIAKI (contrast-induced AKI)
> ✓ Post-angiographic AKI

Figure 2. Multiple naming for post-angiographic AKI. We use post-angiographic AKI in this chapter.

However, contrast media is not a unique cause of AKI after angiography. As discussed below, hemodynamics could cause, or at least modify, the occurrence of AKI after angiography. Therefore, we use post-angiographic AKI, instead of contrast-induced AKI, as a term in this chapter.

Role of Hemodynamics in the Formation of Post-Angiographic AKI; Lessons from Animal Models

Before continuing the discussion of clinical AKI, we would like to brief the pathophysiology of post-angiographic AKI. It is true that there is a species difference between rodent strains and human beings, however, we may find some relevant mechanism from *in vivo* studies. Experimental model of post-angiographic AKI has provided pathophysiological insights. *In vivo* infusion of contrast media resulted in extensive tubular damage with prominent vacuolation (Figure 3) [15-17]. These studies have revealed that kidney parenchyma decreased its partial pressure of oxygen to the critically low levels after the administration of iodinated contrast medium *in vivo* [18].

In addition to this hypoxic toxicity, contrast medium could also directly exert toxicity through reactive oxygen species as seen *in vitro* studies [19-21]. Both hypoxia and reactive oxygen species produce vicious cycle to the acute damage of kidney parenchyma (Figure 4) [18]. Of note, this model requires pre-treatment with both nonsteroidal anti-inflammatory drugs and NO-synthase inhibitors (Figure 4) [17, 18].

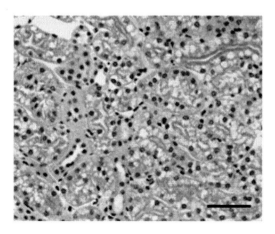

Figure 3. Experimental model of post-angiographic AKI of mouse. Prominent vacuolar changes are seen in the proximal tubules. Scale bars, 50ìm.

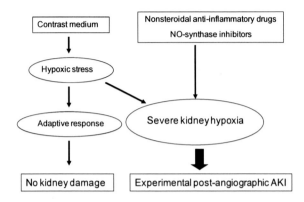

Figure 4. Formation of experimental post-angiographic AKI. *In vivo* infusion of contrast medium results in extensive tubular damage as long as experimental animals are pre-treated with both nonsteroidal anti-inflammatory drugs and NO-synthase inhibitors. Experimental laboratory animals that are subject to contrast media only could adapt to this stress and do not develop AKI. Figure is adapted from [18] with modification.

Table 1. Incidence and risk of post-angiographic AKI

Study, Year (reference)	Population			Outcomes				
	Patients, n	Mean Age, y	Characteristics	Definition of post-angiographic AKI	Incidence of AKI %	Risk of AKI	Odds ratio	95% CI
Levy et al, 1996 [26]*	357	64–68	Angiography	Cre ≥ 25% or to 2 mg/dL	1.1	NR		
McCulbugh et al, 1997 [23]	1826	64	PCI	Cre ≥ 25% Required dialysis	14.5 0.8	Creatinine clearance Diabetes Dose of contrast medium	0.83 5.47 1.008	0.77 – 0.89 1.40 – 21.32 1.002 – 1.013
Gruberg et al,. 2000 [25]	439	70	Cre ≥ 1.8mg/dL PCI	Cre ≥ 25% or required dialysis	37	Blood transfusion Contrast volume Ejection fraction	1.55 1.003 0.97	1.27 – 1.91 1.001 – 1.006 0.95 – 0.99
Rihal et al, 2002 [24]	7586	65	PCI	Cre ≥ 0.5mg/dL	3.3	Age Acute myocardial infarction Cre 2.0–2.9 mg/dL Cre ≥ 3.0mg/dL Contrast volume Diabetes Peripheral vascular disease Right coronary procedure Procedural success	1.02 1.85 7.37 12.82 1.12 1.61 1.71 0.67 0.27	1.01 – 1.03 1.31 – 2.63 4.78 – 11.39 8.01 – 20.54 1.02 – 1.23 1.21 – 2.10 1.23 – 2.37 0.50 – 0.91 0.19 – 0.38
Marenzi et al, 2004 [27]	208	62	PCI	Cre ≥ 0.5mg/dL	19	Age ≥ 75 Anterior myocardial infarction Time-to-reperfusion ≥ 6 hours Contrast volume ≥ 300 mL Usage of intra-aortic balloon pump	5.28 2.17 2.51 2.8 15.51	1.98 – 14.05 0.88 – 5.34 1.01 – 6.16 1.17 – 6.68 4.65 – 51.64
Dangas et al, 2005 [28]	1980	71	PCI CKD	Cre ≥ 25% or Cre ≥ 0.5mg/dL	19.2	eGFR Periprocedural hypotension Pulmonary edema at presentation Usage of intra-aortic balloon pump Ejection fraction less than 40% High contrast volume Hematocrit Diabetes Hypertension	0.97 2.50 2.56 2.27 1.57 1.00 0.95 1.67 1.61	0.96 – 0.98 1.70 – 3.69 1.45 – 4.52 1.29 – 4.00 1.14 – 2.16 1.00 – 1.01 0.92 – 0.97 1.24 – 2.26 1.10 – 2.35
	5250	62	PCI non CKD		13.1	Periprocedural hypotension Pulmonary edema at presentation Ejection fraction less than 40% High contrast volume Hematocrit Diabetes Hypertension Age	2.2 2.68 1.58 1.01 0.95 1.55 1.39 1.03	1.63 – 2.97 1.49 – 4.81 1.24 – 2.01 1.00 – 1.01 0.93 – 0.97 1.26 – 1.91 1.12 – 1.72 1.02 – 1.04
Weisbord et al 2008 [29]	585	69	eGFR < 60 Stable patients	Cre ≥ 0.5mg/dL Cre ≥ 25%	5.3 7.7	NR		

CKD, chronic kidney disease; AKI, acute kidney injury; eGFR, estimated glomerular filtration ratio; PCI, percutaneous coronary artery intervention; NR, not recorded; CI, confidence interval
* Matched-pair analysis.
¶Odds ratio against required dialysis.

In other word, experimental laboratory animals that are subject to contrast media only do not develop AKI. Hypoxia induced by contrast medium alone could invoke cellular adaptive response, resulting in no eminent kidney damage[22]. On the other hand, the pre-treatment, which may mimic clinical predisposition factors, enables post-angiographic AKI in the animal model[18].

Role of Hemodynamics in the Incidence of Post-Angiographic AKI; from the Clinical Points of Views

This experimental model is consistent with the fact that post-angiographic AKI occurs frequently in high-risk patients. Let's turn back to the clinical point of view. Various incidence of post-angiographic AKI has been reported, ranging from 1.1% to 37.7% (Table 1) [23-29]. One main reasons for the varied prevalence and prognosis after AKI is the difference of the studies population. AKI does not occur frequently in hemodynamically stable patients, including computer tomography patients and non-emergent coronary angiography patients, wheras it frequently occurs in studies including hemodynamically unstable patients (Table 1). Studies including hemodynamically unstable patients demonstrated that the incidence of post-angiographic AKI was 3.3% to 37%, and most studies found the incidence more than 10%[23-25]. On the other hand, one study of hemodynamically stable patients demonstrated that relatively low incidence of post-angiographic AKI defined by 50% rise of creatinine (6.5% and 8.5% for patients after computed tomography and coronary angiography, respectively)[29]. We could not compare these studies straightforwardly, because of the difference of AKI definition used, however, there is a tendency that AKI frequently occurs in hemodynamically unstable patients. The identified risk factors of post-angiographic AKI also suggest the implication of hemodynamic instability in the occurrence of AKI. Many risk factors are known in the occurrence of post-angiographic AKI. These factors include diabetes, decreased kidney function, aging, and congestive heart failure[13, 14, 23-25, 28, 30]. They predispose patients to AKI by compromising kidney oxygen supply, worsening kidney microcirculation, or losing the response to vasodilatators. Among these factors, the hemodynamic factors are by far the strongest predictors for post-angiographic AKI[24, 25, 28, 30]. One study found that decreased cardiac function (measured by left ventricular ejection fraction) is the risk of AKI[25]. Another study found that acute myocardial infarction, which is sometimes associated with acute decompensation of hemodynamics, is one of the strong predictors of AKI.[24] Moreover, another study found that periprocedural hypotention, congestive heart failure, usage of intra-aortic ballon pump are by far the strongest predictors of AKI (adjusted odds ratios are 2.50, 2.56, and 2.27, respectively)[28]. One study demonstrated the prediction rule of post-angiograhic AKI[30]. This study independently scored the highest marks to the hemodynamic factors, such as hypotension, usage of intra-aortic balloon pump, and congestive heart failure, to predict post-angiographic AKI (Figure 5)[30]. These studies commonly demonstrated that hemodynamic instability, resulting from congestive heart failure, acute myocardial infarction, periprocedural hypotension, and needing usage of intra-aortic ballon pump or percutaneous cardiopulmonary support, is very strong predictor of AKI.

Table 2. Short-term prognosis of post-angiographic AKI

Study, Year (reference)	Population				Definition of prognosis	Short-term outcomes			
	Patients, n	Mean Age, y	Characteristics	Definition of post-angiographic AKI		Incidence of events, AKI vs non-AKI %		Risk of events Adjusted odds ratio	95% CI
						AKI	non-AKI		
Levy et al, 1996 [26]*	357	64–68		Cre ≥ 25% or to 2 mg/dL	in-hospital mortality	25	9	5.8	2.9 – 13.2
McCulbugh et al, 1997 [23]	1826	64		Cre ≥ 25%	in-hospital mortality	7.1	1.1	NR	
Gruberg et al., 2000 [25]	439	70	Cre ≥ 1.8mg/dL PCI	Cre ≥ 25% or required dialysis	in-hospital mortality	14.9	4.9	NR	
Rhal et al, 2002 [24]	7586	65		Cre ≥ 0.5mg/dL	in-hospital mortality	22.0	1.0	NR	
Marenzi et al, 2004 [27]	208	62		Cre ≥ 0.5mg/dL	in-hospital mortality	31.0	0.6	NR	
Dangas et al, 2005 [28]	1980	71	CKD	Cre ≥ 25% or Cre ≥ 0.5mg/dL	in-hospital mortality	6.3	0.8	NR	
	5250	62	non-CKD			2.5	0.1		
Weisbord et al, 2006 [10]¶	4429	NR	coronary angiography	Cre ≥ 0.25mg/dL	30-days in-hospital mortality	11.2	3.8	1.83	1.4–2.5
				Cre ≥ 0.5mg/dL		16.0	4.2	1.4	0.9–2.3
				Cre ≥ 1.0mg/dL		21.1	4.5	3.0	2.1–1.3
				Cre ≥ 25%		10.4	4.1	1.4	1.0–1.9
				Cre ≥ 50%		19.7	4.2	2.7	1.9–3.8
				Cre ≥ 100%		27.7	4.7	3.6	2.3–5.6
Weisbord et al 2008 [29]	585	69	eGFR < 60 Stable patients undergoing computer tomography and angiography	Cre ≥ 0.5mg/dL Cre ≥ 25%	30-days in-hospital mortality	NR		7.0	1.0–40.1
								3.9	0.6–20.3

CKD, chronic kidney disease; AKI, acute kidney injury; NR, not recorded; CI, confidence interval
* Matched-pair analysis.
¶ Patients with measured creatinine were collected from 20,866 patients.

However, these too strong odds ratios may indicate that these hemodynamic factors are involved in the pathogenesis of AKI, rather than they are independent predictors of AKI[31].

The results of these studies, along with the results of experimental models, indicate that post-angiographic AKI occurs mainly in hemodynamically unstable patients.

Short-Term Prognosis of Post-Angiographic AKI

Besides the incidence, the prognosis of AKI patients is of great interest for clinicians, and we hint on one question; whether post-angiographic AKI in itself has impact on prognosis, or whether AKI, in conjugation with hemodynamic instability, has the impact. We need to understand the result of clinical studies, taking hemodynamic instability into consideration. It is evident that acute hemodynamic instability described above has a strong impact not only on the incidence of AKI, but also on the prognosis[31-34]. Recent studies have demonstrated that patients experiencing post-angiographic AKI have a greater risk of in-hospital mortality (Table 2)[10, 13, 23-25, 27, 28]. One study demonstrated in-hospital mortality was 14.9% and 4.9% for AKI and non-AKI patients, respectively[25]. If multiple logistic regression analyses had been performed in these studies, we assume that AKI would be selected as a strong predictor of in-hospital mortality. However, to examine the impact of AKI on the short-term outcomes is extremely difficult. In other word, simple adjustment may not be sufficient to determine the cause-and-effect relationship[12, 31]. Hemodynamically unstable patients were substantially included in post-angiographic AKI patients, and the cause of hemodynamic instability may persist even after the angiography (Figure 6). As a result, these patients may die because the hemodynamic instability has persisted after angiography (Figure 6). It is difficult to determine the cause of death in those who died from AKI or from hemodynamic instability.

Risk factors	Integer score
Hypotension	5
Intra-aortic ballon pump	5
Congestive heart failure	5
Age ≥ 75	4
Anemia	3
Diabetes	3
Volume of contrast medium	1 for 100 mL
eGFR 40-60	2
eGFR 20-40	4
eGFR < 20	6

summed →

Risk score	Risk of AKI, %
≤ 5	0.075
6 - 10	14
11 - 16	26.1
≥ 16	57.3

Figure 5. Scheme to define AKI risk score after percutaneous coronary intervention. AKI risk stratification score based on 8 variables was provided. Risk score is obtained by summing integer score. Figure is adapted from [30] with modification.

Therefore, it looks rather reasonable to study the short-term impact of AKI in hemodynamic stable population, however, this design of study still has a problem. One prospective study examined relatively stable 165 patients (outpatient undergoing computer tomography)[35]. They found that incidence of AKI was 6.1-8.5%, depending on the definition of AKI, and only one patient died within 30 days. 38 patients re-hospitalized within 30 days, however, AKI was not associated with the short-term re-hospitalization. As a result, they could not determine the impact of AKI on the short-term prognosis because of extremely low incidence of AKI[35]. Even if one studies the impact of AKI on the short-term prognosis of stable patients in the larger cohort, it would be very difficult to find the association between AKI and prognosis because of the extremely low incidence of hard outcomes (death or cardiovascular events). The low incidence of outcome may also indicate that there is not a big benefit in the intervention to stable patients. We hesitate to study the short-term impact of AKI for these reasons. What we could draw the conclusion from the result of previous studies is that AKI may represent the existence of high risk factors, i.e., hemodynamic instability. AKI could be used a surrogate marker of the short-term outcomes. In other word, we still have not enough evidence that usage of contrast medium in itself is the risk of the short-term outcomes.

Long-Term Prognosis and Post-Angiographic AKI: Role of Hemodynamics

The next question we came across is whether post-angiographic AKI alone has impact on the long-term prognosis, or whether AKI, in conjugation with hemodynamic disturbance, has the impact[12]. Previous studies have identified post-angiographic AKI as a strong predictor of the long-term prognosis[13, 14, 23, 25, 28, 36]. On the other hand, hemodynamic factors have also been selected as very strong predictors of the long-term mortality in these studies (Table 3) [25, 28]. One study of CKD patients demonstrated that adjusted odds ratio of post-angiographic AKI for one-year mortality was 2.37 (95% CI, 1.63 -3.44), while those of hemodynamic variables were extremely high (adjusted odds ratios [95% CI] for hypotension, usage of intra-aortic balloon pump, ejection fraction below 40% were 3.18 [2.08 – 4.86], 2.49 [1.41 – 4.41], and 1.66 [1.15 – 2.41], respectively)[28]. In order to explore impact of AKI in itself, not hemodynamic factor, on the long-term prognosis, we performed analysis as below. We planed to analyze the impact of post-angiographic AKI on the long-term prognosis in whole population and in hemodynamically stable group. We did not analyze this in hemodynamically unstable patients for several reasons; i) the cohort only included relatively small number of hemodynamically unstable patients, and ii) the degree of hemodynamic instability varied widely in these patients, and we could not regard them as homogeneously "hemodynamically unstable". On selecting hemodynamically stable population, we first thought of studying patients undergoing angiographic computed tomography in the outpatient settings. One study performed the incidence of AKI in such population[37]. They demonstrated that the incidence of AKI is infrequent in CKD outpatients (3.6% for the rise of creatinine more than 25%). The long-term prognositic analysis of such patients is not realistic because this will need extremely high number and long observational period. Therefore, we analyzed historical cohort of coronary angiographic population.

Table 3. Long-term prognosis of post-angiographic AKI

Study, Year (reference)	Population Patients, n	Mean Age, y	Characteristics	Definition of post-angiographic AKI	Inclusion of in-hospital mortality outcomes	Definition of outcomes	Incidence of events, AKI vs non-AKI, % 0.5 year	1 year	3 year	5 year	Long-term outcomes Adjusted risk	Risk score	95% CI
Gruberg et al. 2000 [25]*	439	70	Cre ≥ 1.8mg/dL	Cre ≥ 25% or required dialysis	Yes	Mortality		37.7 19.4			AKI Age Vein graft lesion location	3.86 1.05 1.55	1.96-7.58 1.05-1.09 0.95-2.52
Rihal et al. 2002 [24]	7586	65		Cre ≥ 0.5mg/dL	No	Mortality		12.1 3.7		44.6 14.5	NR		
Dangas et al. 2005 [28]*	2005		CKD	Cre ≥ 25% or Cre ≥ 0.5mg/dL	Yes	Mortality		22.6 6.9			AKI Hypotension Intra-aortic balloon pumping Ejection fraction < 40% Peripheral vascular disease Diabetes eGFR Older age	2.37 3.18 2.49 1.66 1.85 1.92 0.97 1.03	1.63-3.44 2.08-4.86 1.41-4.41 1.15-2.41 1.30-2.65 1.34-2.76 0.96-0.99 1.01-1.05
	5543		non-CKD					8.0 2.7			AKI Hypotension Intra-aortic balloon pumping Ejection fraction < 40% Peripheral vascular disease Diabetes Older age History of stroke Hematocrit	1.86 2.70 2.04 3.26 1.78 1.56 1.03 1.55 0.90	1.27-2.74 1.76-4.14 1.11-3.76 2.32-4.58 1.23-2.59 1.12-2.19 1.01-1.04 1.01-2.39 0.86-0.93
Solomon et al. 2009 [36] ¶	294		CKD	Cre ≥ 0.3mg/dL	NR	Combination of death, stroke, myocardial infarction, or ESRD		43 29			AKI	3.2	1.1-8.7
Kimura et al. 2010 [12]	2439	66.3	CKD	Cre ≥ 25% or Cre ≥ 0.3mg/dL	No	Mortality Whole population	2.7 1.1	4.1 1.9	11.0 4.8	20.2 8.2			
						Stable population	2.0 1.0	4.0 1.7	6.7 4.4	6.7 7.9			
						Combination of death and cardiovascular events Whole population	14.5 4.0	18.8 6.7	35.6 11.2	41.1 18.4			
						Stable population	9.4 4.0	15.6 6.4	25.4 10.8	33.5 18.1			

CKD, chronic kidney disease; AKI, acute kidney injury; eGFR, estimated glomerular filtration rate; NR, not recorded; CI, confidence interval
*Odds ratios for one-year mortality were calculated.
¶Incidence rate ratio for one-year mortality was calculated.

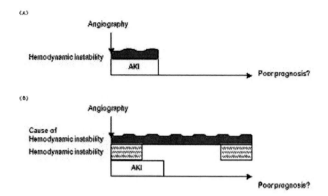

Figure 6. The relationship between post-angiographic AKI, hemodynamic instability, and prognosis. At the moment, it seems uncertain whether AKI in itself affects prognosis (A) or whether AKI in conjugation with the cause of hemodynamic instability (B), affects through AKI.

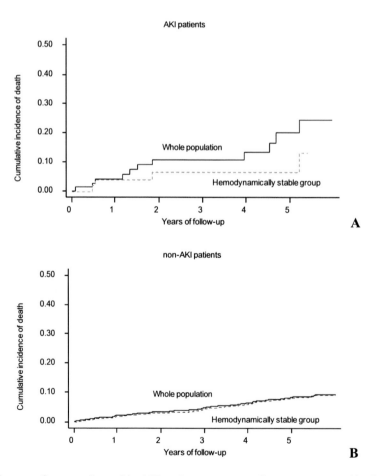

Figure 7. The impact of post-angiographic AKI on long-term mortality was attenuated in the hemodynamically stable population. Kaplan-Meier curve seen in the analysis of all patients was attenuated in the hemodynamically stable group of AKI patients (A), while the curve of all patients was not in the hemodynamically stable group of non-AKI patients (B). Solid line, whole population, dotted line, hemodynamically stable group.

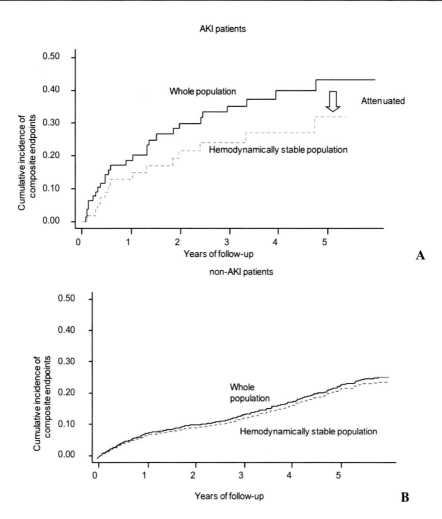

Figure 8. The impact of post-angiographic AKI on long-term composite end points was attenuated in the hemodynamically stable population. Kaplan-Meier curve seen in the analysis of all patients was attenuated in the hemodynamically stable group of AKI patients (A), while the curve of all patients was not in the hemodynamically stable group of non-AKI patients (B). Solid line, whole population, dotted line, hemodynamically stable group.

We studied 2,439 patients who underwent coronary angiography or percutaneous coronary intervention. AKI was defined as proposed by the Acute Kidney Injury Network (an absolute increase of at least 0.3 mg/dL or 50 % from the baseline serum creatinine within 48 hours)[1]. We defined patients presenting with hypotension (systolic blood pressure below 80 mmHg), using the intra-aortic balloon pump and/or percutaneous cardiopulmonary support, intubated into trachea due to pulmonary congestion, or using catecholamine, as hemodynamically unstable.

We started our observation after the discharge from the index hospital stay mainly for the reasons below. First, it is difficult to differentiate patients who die from AKI from those who die from any other event (mainly the disease for which they are admitted to hospital). Second, in-hospital death occurred within a short period at the beginning. The number of deaths was not small, however, and we are concerned about the possibility that the Cox proportionality assumption may be violated if we include them in the model. In our analysis, the assumption of Cox proportionality is not violated.

The final analysis covered 2,193 patients with a mean age of 66.3 ± 11.4 years and the mean eGFR was 72.1 ± 21.5 mL/$1.73m^2$. Incidence of AKI was 3.7%. Follow-up ratio was relatively good for retrospective study; 74.1% for death and 75.4% for composite end point. We attributed this to the well-achieved regional partnership with primary care physicians and specificity of the studied region. Univariate Cox regression analysis revealed that post-angiographic AKI was a predictor of both mortality (HR [95% CI]; 2.61 [1.44 to 4.71]) and composite end point (defined as mortality and cardiovascular events, HR [95% CI] 2.59 [1.78 to 3.78], Table 4). The relationship of post-angiographic AKI and composite end point persisted after adjustment for other comorbidities (adjusted HR [95% CI] 1.64 [1.09 to 2.46]).

We performed Kaplan-Meier analysis in whole patients and in the hemodynamically stable patients (Figure 7,8). These curves demonstrated that the impact of AKI in the analysis of all patients could be attenuated in hemodynamically stable group. Multivariable analysis of hemodynamically stable group revealed AKI was not a predictor of both mortality (AHR [95% CI] 0.97 [0.39 to 2.45]) and composite end point (1.32 [0.79 to 2.23]). Our result suggested that, among hospital survivors, the impact of AKI on hemodynamically stable patients was attenuated compared with that in our overall patient population.

The result of our study should be understood within the limitations of the methodology adopted. We started observation after the discharges of patients, in contrast with previous studies, which began their observation from the index hospital stay.Therefore, very high-risk patients who died during the hospital stay were excluded from our cohort. This results in the lower incidence of AKI and lower mortality of our cohort. Our finding could not be externally validated in the impact of post-angiographic AKI on the short-term outcomes.As described above, although negative impact of AKI on in-hospital mortality has been implied, however, the precise impact remains to be assessed. Furthermore, we were unable to analyze the long-term impact of AKI on hemodynamically unstable patients because of the small number and inhomogeneous character of such patients.The wide confidence intervals of our findings and the nature of our cohort (historical cohort) made it impossible to definitively determine the impact of AKI on the long-term prognosis in our hemodynamically stable patients.

Even after taking these limitations into account, our result suggests that the impact of AKI on long-term prognosis may be attenuated in hemodynamically stable hospital survivors.

Table 4. The long-term impact of post-angiographic AKI

End point	Whole population				Hemodynamically stable patients			
	Unadjusted model		Multivariable model[a]		Unadjusted model		Multivariable model[b]	
Death from any cause	2.61	(1.44 – 4.71)	1.53	(0.84 – 2.91)	1.58	(0.64 – 3.85)	0.97	(0.39 – 2.45)
Composite end point	2.59	(1.78 – 3.78)	1.64	(1.09 – 2.46)	1.94	(1.18 – 3.20)	1.32	(0.79 – 2.23)

Values are described as HR (95%CI).
[a] Models were developed by adjustment with clinically relevant parameters.
[b] Models were developed with the variables as in model a, except for hemodynamic instability.

Role of Contrast Media in the Formation of Future Post-Angiographic AKI

We believe that the impact of contrast media in itself on the occurrence of AKI has been reduced remarkably these days, and will be reduced further, for two reasons (Figure 9). First, the type of contrast medium has been improved to be lower in osmolarity and viscosity. Contrast medium is known for its high osmolarity and viscosity, and this property has been implied as the cause of AKI.

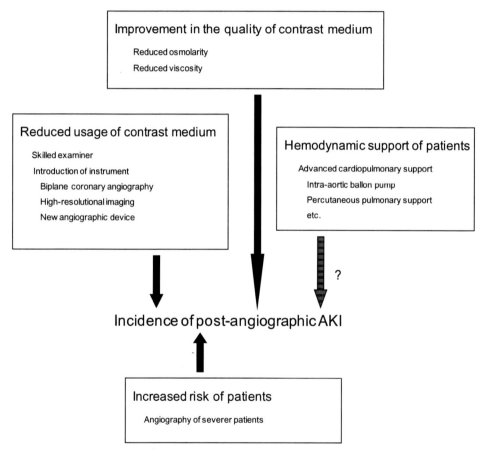

Figure 9. Reduced impact of contrast medium in the occurrence of post-angiographic AKI. The impact of contrast media in itself on the occurrence of AKI has been reduced remarkably these days, and will be reduced further through presented mechanism. The type of contrast medium has much been improved to be lower in osmolarity and viscosity. Newer medium has been remarkably improved in their osmolarity and viscosity, which will potentially reduce the risk of AKI. The dose of contrast medium used in angiography has been remarkably lowered by the effort of examiner and by the improvement of the instruments. The prevalence of biplane coronary angiography, along with high-resolution x-ray angiography, innovation of angiographic devices and improvement of examiners' skill, has remarkably reduced the dose of contrast media. Intensive hemodynamic support during angiography may reduce the incidence of AKI by keeping kidney blood perfusion. On the other hand, the number of angiography of severer cases may increase, and this could result in the increased incidence of post-angiographic AKI.

However, newer medium has been remarkably improved in their osmolarity and viscosity, which will potentially reduce the risk. Second, the dose of contrast medium used in angiography has been remarkably lowered by the effort of examiner and by the improvement of the instruments. The prevalence of biplane coronary angiography, along with high-resolution x-ray angiography, innovation of angiographic devices and improvement of examiners' skill, has remarkably reduced the dose of contrast media. As a result, some angiographic procedures, which took several hundreds mL of contrast media, only need less than 20 mL. Intensive hemodynamic support during angiography may reduce the incidence of AKI by keeping kidney blood perfusion. Angiographic procedure these days needs smaller and smaller amount of contrast medium. On the other hand, the cases which need large amount of contrast medium (for example, more than 300 mL) may possess severe artery lesions or poor in hemodynamic condition. The severe lesions and poor hemodynamical conditions are associated with poor prognosis by themselves.

Conclusion

Post-angiographic AKI should be studied, not only from the point of direct effect of contrast medium, but also from the point of hemodynamics. We are not certain which has more impact, however, at least we now know that both of them are deeply involved in the prognosis after post-angiographic AKI. Future studies should aim to clarify the relationship of these factors.

References

[1]   Mehta RL, Kellum JA, Shah SV, Molitoris BA, Ronco C, Warnock DG, et al. Acute Kidney Injury Network: report of an initiative to improve outcomes in acute kidney injury. *Crit. Care.* 2007;11(2):R31.
[2]   Bellomo R, Ronco C, Kellum JA, Mehta RL, Palevsky P. Acute renal failure - definition, outcome measures, animal models, fluid therapy and information technology needs: the Second International Consensus Conference of the Acute Dialysis Quality Initiative (ADQI) Group. *Crit. Care.* 2004 Aug;8(4):R204-12.
[3]   Clermont G, Acker CG, Angus DC, Sirio CA, Pinsky MR, Johnson JP. Renal failure in the ICU: comparison of the impact of acute renal failure and end-stage renal disease on ICU outcomes. *Kidney Int.* 2002 Sep;62(3):986-96.
[4]   Mehta RL, Pascual MT, Soroko S, Savage BR, Himmelfarb J, Ikizler TA, et al. Spectrum of acute renal failure in the intensive care unit: the PICARD experience. *Kidney Int.* 2004 Oct;66(4):1613-21.
[5]   Metnitz PG, Krenn CG, Steltzer H, Lang T, Ploder J, Lenz K, et al. Effect of acute renal failure requiring renal replacement therapy on outcome in critically ill patients. *Crit. Care Med.* 2002 Sep;30(9):2051-8.
[6]   Uchino S, Kellum JA, Bellomo R, Doig GS, Morimatsu H, Morgera S, et al. Acute renal failure in critically ill patients: a multinational, multicenter study. *JAMA.* 2005 Aug 17;294(7):813-8.

[7]   Chertow GM, Burdick E, Honour M, Bonventre JV, Bates DW. Acute kidney injury, mortality, length of stay, and costs in hospitalized patients. *J. Am. Soc. Nephrol.* 2005 Nov;16(11):3365-70.

[8]   Forman DE, Butler J, Wang Y, Abraham WT, O'Connor CM, Gottlieb SS, et al. Incidence, predictors at admission, and impact of worsening renal function among patients hospitalized with heart failure. *J. Am. Coll. Cardiol.* 2004 Jan 7;43(1):61-7.

[9]   Parikh CR, Coca SG, Wang Y, Masoudi FA, Krumholz HM. Long-term prognosis of acute kidney injury after acute myocardial infarction. *Arch. Intern. Med.* 2008 May 12;168(9):987-95.

[10] Weisbord SD, Chen H, Stone RA, Kip KE, Fine MJ, Saul MI, et al. Associations of increases in serum creatinine with mortality and length of hospital stay after coronary angiography. *J. Am. Soc. Nephrol.* 2006 Oct;17(10):2871-7.

[11] Coca SG, Yusuf B, Shlipak MG, Garg AX, Parikh CR. Long-term risk of mortality and other adverse outcomes after acute kidney injury: a systematic review and meta-analysis. *Am. J. Kidney Dis.* 2009 Jun;53(6):961-73.

[12] Kimura T, Obi Y, Yasuda K, Sasaki KI, Takeda Y, Nagai Y, et al. Effects of chronic kidney disease and post-angiographic acute kidney injury on long-term prognosis after coronary artery angiography. *Nephrol. Dial. Transplant.* 2010 Oct 12.

[13] Barrett BJ, Parfrey PS. Clinical practice. Preventing nephropathy induced by contrast medium. *N. Engl. J. Med.* 2006 Jan 26;354(4):379-86.

[14] McCullough PA. Contrast-induced acute kidney injury. *J. Am. Coll. Cardiol.* 2008 Apr 15;51(15):1419-28.

[15] Heyman SN, Reichman J, Brezis M. Pathophysiology of radiocontrast nephropathy: a role for medullary hypoxia. *Invest. Radiol.* 1999 Nov;34(11):685-91.

[16] Heyman SN, Brezis M, Epstein FH, Spokes K, Silva P, Rosen S. Early renal medullary hypoxic injury from radiocontrast and indomethacin. *Kidney Int.* 1991 Oct;40(4):632-42.

[17] Billings FTt, Chen SW, Kim M, Park SW, Song JH, Wang S, et al. alpha2-Adrenergic agonists protect against radiocontrast-induced nephropathy in mice. *Am. J. Physiol. Renal Physiol.* 2008 Sep;295(3):F741-8.

[18] Heyman SN, Rosen S, Rosenberger C. Renal parenchymal hypoxia, hypoxia adaptation, and the pathogenesis of radiocontrast nephropathy. *Clin. J. Am. Soc. Nephrol.* 2008 Jan;3(1):288-96.

[19] Haller C, Hizoh I. The cytotoxicity of iodinated radiocontrast agents on renal cells in vitro. *Invest. Radiol.* 2004 Mar;39(3):149-54.

[20] Bakris GL, Lass N, Gaber AO, Jones JD, Burnett JC, Jr. Radiocontrast medium-induced declines in renal function: a role for oxygen free radicals. *Am. J. Physiol.* 1990 Jan;258(1 Pt 2):F115-20.

[21] Zager RA, Johnson AC, Hanson SY. Radiographic contrast media-induced tubular injury: evaluation of oxidant stress and plasma membrane integrity. *Kidney Int.* 2003 Jul;64(1):128-39.

[22] Rosenberger C, Heyman SN, Rosen S, Shina A, Goldfarb M, Griethe W, et al. Up-regulation of HIF in experimental acute renal failure: evidence for a protective transcriptional response to hypoxia. *Kidney Int.* 2005 Feb;67(2):531-42.

[23] McCullough PA, Wolyn R, Rocher LL, Levin RN, O'Neill WW. Acute renal failure after coronary intervention: incidence, risk factors, and relationship to mortality. *Am. J. Med.* 1997 Nov;103(5):368-75.

[24] Rihal CS, Textor SC, Grill DE, Berger PB, Ting HH, Best PJ, et al. Incidence and prognostic importance of acute renal failure after percutaneous coronary intervention. *Circulation.* 2002 May 14;105(19):2259-64.

[25] Gruberg L, Mintz GS, Mehran R, Gangas G, Lansky AJ, Kent KM, et al. The prognostic implications of further renal function deterioration within 48 h of interventional coronary procedures in patients with pre-existent chronic renal insufficiency. *J. Am. Coll. Cardiol.* 2000 Nov 1;36(5):1542-8.

[26] Levy EM, Viscoli CM, Horwitz RI. The effect of acute renal failure on mortality. A cohort analysis. *JAMA.* 1996 May 15;275(19):1489-94.

[27] Marenzi G, Lauri G, Assanelli E, Campodonico J, De Metrio M, Marana I, et al. Contrast-induced nephropathy in patients undergoing primary angioplasty for acute myocardial infarction. *J. Am. Coll. Cardiol.* 2004 Nov 2;44(9):1780-5.

[28] Dangas G, Iakovou I, Nikolsky E, Aymong ED, Mintz GS, Kipshidze NN, et al. Contrast-induced nephropathy after percutaneous coronary interventions in relation to chronic kidney disease and hemodynamic variables. *Am. J. Cardiol.* 2005 Jan 1;95(1):13-9.

[29] Weisbord SD, Mor MK, Resnick AL, Hartwig KC, Sonel AF, Fine MJ, et al. Prevention, incidence, and outcomes of contrast-induced acute kidney injury. *Arch. Intern. Med.* 2008 Jun 23;168(12):1325-32.

[30] Mehran R, Aymong ED, Nikolsky E, Lasic Z, Iakovou I, Fahy M, et al. A simple risk score for prediction of contrast-induced nephropathy after percutaneous coronary intervention: development and initial validation. *J. Am. Coll. Cardiol.* 2004 Oct 6;44(7):1393-9.

[31] Rudnick M, Feldman H. Contrast-induced nephropathy: what are the true clinical consequences? *Clin. J. Am. Soc. Nephrol.* 2008 Jan;3(1):263-72.

[32] Haft JW, Pagani FD, Romano MA, Leventhal CL, Dyke DB, Matthews JC. Short- and long-term survival of patients transferred to a tertiary care center on temporary extracorporeal circulatory support. *Ann. Thorac. Surg.* 2009 Sep;88(3):711-7; discussion 7-8.

[33] Jaski BE, Lingle RJ, Overlie P, Favrot LK, Willms DC, Chillcott S, et al. Long-term survival with use of percutaneous extracorporeal life support in patients presenting with acute myocardial infarction and cardiovascular collapse. *ASAIO J.* 1999 Nov-Dec;45(6):615-8.

[34] Sprung J, Ritter MJ, Rihal CS, Warner ME, Wilson GA, Williams BA, et al. Outcomes of cardiopulmonary resuscitation and predictors of survival in patients undergoing coronary angiography including percutaneous coronary interventions. *Anesth. Analg.* 2006 Jan;102(1):217-24.

[35] Weisbord SD, Hartwig KC, Sonel AF, Fine MJ, Palevsky P. The incidence of clinically significant contrast-induced nephropathy following non-emergent coronary angiography. *Catheter Cardiovasc. Interv.* 2008 Jun 1;71(7):879-85.

[36] Solomon RJ, Mehran R, Natarajan MK, Doucet S, Katholi RE, Staniloae CS, et al. Contrast-induced nephropathy and long-term adverse events: cause and effect? *Clin. J. Am. Soc. Nephrol.* 2009 Jul;4(7):1162-9.

[37] Weisbord SD, Mor MK, Resnick AL, Hartwig KC, Palevsky PM, Fine MJ. Incidence and outcomes of contrast-induced AKI following computed tomography. *Clin. J. Am. Soc. Nephrol.* 2008 Sep;3(5):1274-81.

In: Acute Kidney Injury: Causes, Diagnosis and Treatments   ISBN: 978-1-61209-790-9
Editor: Jonathan D. Mendoza, pp. 69-88   © 2011 Nova Science Publishers, Inc.

Chapter V

Cardiac Surgery-Associated Acute Kidney Injury

Vijaykumar Lingegowda[*], *Mourad Alsabbagh, and A. Ahsan Ejaz*
Division of Nephrology, Hypertension and Transplantation,
University of Florida, Gainesville, Florida, USA

Introduction

Acute kidney injury (AKI) is a serious complication of cardiac surgery. Cardiac surgery-associated AKI (CSA-AKI) is associated with high in-hospital mortality, complicated hospital course, a high risk of infectious complications and high utilization of resources. The spectrum of CSA-AKI can range from subclinical renal injury to severe AKI requiring Renal Replacement Therapy (RRT). Patients with AKI requiring RRT have 30-day mortality rates in excess of 40%. Despite the advances in bypass techniques, intensive care, and delivery of RRT, mortality and morbidity associated with AKI have not changed much in recent years. Even small increases in serum creatinine (SCr) after surgery, that is not associated with need for RRT, are also associated with significantly increased risk of mortality, both in the short and long-term. The normalization of elevated serum creatinine prior to discharge from the hospital does not appear to reduce the risk of increased mortality in these patients. There is however, considerable heterogeneity in the mortality rates in different studies due to the lack of uniform criteria for the definition of AKI. Herein we discuss the proposed pathomechanisms of CSA-AKI and recent strategies for diagnosis and prevention of CSA-AKI.

[*] Corresponding author: Vijaykumar Lingegowda, M.D., MSEd, Division of Nephrology, Hypertension and Transplantation, University of Florida, P.O. Box 100224, Gainesville, FL 32610-0224, U.S.A. Tel: 702-518-5418, Fax: 352-392-3581 , Email: vgowda2@yahoo.com

Epidemiology

The incidence of CSA-AKI varies according to the definition utilized in any particular study. Estimating the incidence becomes more complicated when one considers that more than thirty different definitions of AKI have been reported in the literature. In one study where AKI was defined as a rise in serum creatinine of > 1mg/dl above baseline, the incidence of CSA-AKI was reported to be 8%, and the incidence of AKI requiring RRT was 0.7% [1]. The incidence of CSA-AKI also varies with the severity of baseline cardiac and renal function and types of cardiac surgery performed. Although data are limited, patients with preexisting chronic kidney disease are at higher risk for CSA-AKI than those with normal preoperative kidney function. The risk for CSA-AKI is also much higher in patients undergoing thoracic aortic aneurysm surgery compared to those undergoing cardiac valve or coronary artery bypass surgery [2,3]. When AKI is defined as requirement for dialysis, the incidence of CSA-AKI is 1-5% [1,4-15].

Multiple studies have shown that mortality is high in patients who develop CSA-AKI versus those who do not, and the mortality rates vary from 15-60% depending on the definition of AKI used and duration of follow up [1, 4-15]. In patients who develop CSA-AKI requiring RRT, mortality rates have been reported in excess of 50% in most of the studies reported [1, 4-15]. Another consistent finding across many studies is that even mild elevation of serum creatinine after the surgery is associated with significant increase in mortality and return of creatinine back to baseline before discharge does not seem to reduce this risk. Studies by Lassnigg et al. have demonstrated that the 30-day mortality was 2.5-fold higher in patients who developed a 0-0.5mg/dl rise in creatinine postoperatively compared to those who did not have any rise; and the mortality was more than 18-fold higher in those who had a creatinine rise of > 0.5mg/dl [16]. Similarly, postoperative decline in estimated glomerular filtration rate was also associated with an increase in 30-day mortality [17].

CSA-AKI is associated with increased cost and utilization of scarce health-care resources. Dasta et al. have reported that the intensive care unit and postoperative-care related costs and average length of stay for patients with AKI are higher than matched controls and these values increase as CSA-AKI severity worsens. In fact the average difference in total postoperative costs between the three RIFLE categories was ~USD 9,000 to 14, 000 [18]. These numbers are in line with a previous study done by Mangano et al. which reported that patients with renal impairment incurred higher ICU (1.7-fold), pharmacy (2.3-fold) and laboratory costs (1.6-fold) compared to controls [4].

Risk Factors for CSA-AKI

Multiple studies have been done and various models have been developed over the years to predict the patient population more likely to develop AKI following cardiac surgery. Chertow et al. [19] developed one of the first models and since then many other groups have developed scoring systems to predict CSA-AKI [1, 20-21]. The risk factors for AKI following cardiac surgery can be broadly divided in to patient-associated factors and procedure-related factors. The patient related risk factors include advanced age, female gender, diabetes, congestive heart failure, low cardiac index, preexisting chronic kidney disease, peripheral vascular disease, chronic obstructive pulmonary disease, preoperative use of balloon pump (cardiogenic shock) and need for more complex or valvular surgery [42,43]. These risk factors have been validated across most of the studies [1, 19, 20-22,42-46]. Among the patient-related risk factors, the strongest and most validated is preoperative creatinine (preexisting renal disease). The risk of AKI requiring Hemodialysis (HD) is about 10-20% in patients with a preoperative baseline creatinine of 2.0-4.0 and 25-28% in patients with a baseline creatinine of >4.0 [19, 20,23-26]. The procedure-related risk factors are more controversial, however are potentially modifiable. They include total duration of CardioPulmonary Bypass (CPB), pulsatile versus non-pulsatile flow, on versus off- pump coronary bypass procedures and normothermic versus hypothermic bypass surgery [27-41]. Among procedure-related risk factors off pump coronary artery bypass is most controversial. Although it removes the need for bypass circuit it is associated with greater hemodynamic instability [38]. The data on this issue is still not quite clear however available evidence is in favor of off pump bypass, especially in patients with preexisting kidney disease [41, 46-48].

Pathophysiology

There are multiple mechanisms by which renal injury occurs during a cardiac surgery. The four major proposed pathways are: hypoperfusion leading to ischemia-reperfusion injury, systemic inflammatory response syndrome (SIRS), embolic injury, and exogenous and endogenous toxins.

Hypoperfusion

Although kidney receives a large portion of cardiac output, majority of the blood flow goes to renal cortex which has a low oxygen extraction ratio. The renal medulla receives a lower proportion of renal blood flow and has higher oxygen consumption. This heterogeneous distribution of blood and consumption of oxygen makes renal medulla highly vulnerable to hypoxia during the periods of hypoperfusion. Hypoperfusion and associated hypoxia leads to series of events that eventually lead to cellular injury [49-53]. Initially hypoxia leads to ATP depletion and oxidative injury. Subsequently there is activation of bone marrow-derived cells, endothelial cells, and renal epithelial cells leading to proinflammatory state. Inflammatory cells adhere to activated endothelium in peritubular capillaries leading to medullary congestion and further hypoxic injury to proximal tubule. Furthermore elaboration of proinflammatory cytokines leads to additional cellular injury.

Patients undergoing cardiac surgery are at high risk for hypoperfusion during preoperative period, CPB time and immediate postoperative period (post-CPB). In the preoperative period patients may have reduced renal perfusion secondary to poor cardiac function (myocardial infarction, valvular disease or cardiogenic shock) which may be further exacerbated by use of diuretics, Angiotensin Converting Enzyme Inhibitors (ACE-I), or Angiotensin Receptor Blockers (ARB). The intra-operative phase is even more critical when patients are exposed to anesthesia and cardiopulmonary bypass. In most centers cardio-pulmonary bypass is accomplished using non-pulsatile pumps. Even if flow from the pump is maintained at the level of normal cardiac output (2.2-2.4L/min/m2), the mean pressures may be lower than normal mean pressures [45]. It is likely that renal perfusion and autoregulation are maintained at these pressures although they are minimal blood flow needed to support organ function. Even small variation in flow from this would likely lead to hypoperfusion and organ damage. This balance is even more delicate in patients with preexisting renal disease and impaired autoregulation specifically patients with prolonged history of high blood pressure. Most centers employ mild to moderate hypothermia during CPB to provide protection against hypoperfusion-related ischemia [45]. Low perfusion flows (for example, 0.5 l/min/m2) or periods of circulatory arrest may be necessary [45] which further enhances the chances of renal injury. Transition from full cardio-pulmonary support with CPB to patient's own cardiovascular system may sometimes be associated with marked hemodynamic instability. During this period patients are at risk for cardiogenic and non-cardiogenic shock, which may further impair the renal perfusion and increase the likelihood of ischemic injury to the kidneys.

Systemic Inflammatory Response Syndrome

Cardiac surgery under CPB causes SIRS due to surgical trauma, contact of blood with foreign materials, abnormal shear stress, ischemia, reperfusion, hypothermia, and unphysiological situations [54]. SIRS occurring after cardiac surgery is associated with massive, unbalanced induction of cytokines [54]. Study done by Hirai showed high circulating levels of inflammatory cytokines IL 6 and IL-8 from 1 hour to 3 hours after removal of cross clamps and longer CPB time showed severe elevation of circulating cytokines [54]. IL-8 induces the amplification of neutrophils and macrophages [44] and has been thought to regulate neutrophil transendothelial migration and potentially control neutrophil mediated tissue injury [54]. Both neutrophils and vascular endothelium are activated with up regulation of adhesion molecules such as CD-11b and CD-41 [47, 55-57]. This results in migration and accumulation of leucocytes in vascular endothelial cells and ultimately may lead to organ damage. Platelets also undergo activation, degranulation and adherence to vascular endothelium [56-58]. There is also an increased production of anti-inflammatory cytokine IL-10, which may be an attempt by the host to counteract the effects of inflammatory cytokines IL-6 and IL-8. Ultimately the relative balance between the proinflammatory and anti-inflammatory cytokines would determine the extent on organ damage [54].

Embolic Injury

During CPB the stream of blood from the arterial cannula can dislodge plaques from aorta, which may embolize in to variety of sites including the kidneys leading to kidney injury. If femoral arterial cannulation is used, plaques can be raised by the retrograde blood stream, and debris directed proximally, particularly to the renal, mesenteric, and cerebral circulations [45]. Emboli or small pieces of vegetations from interior of the heart specially left ventricle or left atrium may also get dislodged and get into systemic circulation during the surgery. Air may also enter the heart through left sided incision during aortic or mitral valve surgery, or during cannulation of left atrium, ventricle or pulmonary veins and if not completely removed before heart begins to eject may lead to distal emboli including emboli to renal circulation.

Exogenous and Endogenous Toxins

Cardiac surgery patients are usually exposed to several medications some of which can be nephrotoxic. These include antibiotics mainly beta-lactams, aminoglycosides or vancomycin among others which can cause neprhotoxicity in variety of mechanisms depending on the drug used. Most of these patients are already on ACEI or ARBs which are able to cause renal damage in some group of patients. They may have also had recent coronary angiogram or other radiological procedures requiring intravenous contrast.

CPB specially if prolonged is associated with the generation of free hemoglobin through hemolysis which may be due to cardiotomy suction, occlusive roller pumps, turbulent flow in the oxygenator, and blood return through cell savers [46]. In the presence of oxidants such as hydrogen peroxide and superoxide, free low molecular mass iron is released from the heme moiety into circulation [59]. This is able to participate in organic and inorganic oxygen radical reactions including lipid peroxidation and formation of hydroxyl radicals with subsequent tissue damage [60]. Splanchnic hypoperfusion during CPB or post CPB is believed to cause endotoxemia which could contribute to renal injury [61].

Others

Plasma levels of hormones such as epinephrine, norepineprhine, dopamine and vasopressin rise during CPB. These changes lead to reduction in renal blood flow, and concomitant reduction in GFR.

Diagnosis

The prevailing weakness with the CSA-AKI definitions is that it is still based on an increase in SCr or decrease in urine volume. SCr and Blood Urea Nitrogen (BUN) have been used to monitor kidney dysfunction for over a century but these markers are insensitive and non-specific [62]. SCr is dependent not only on GFR but also on many other factors such as, rate of tubular secretion of creatinine, rate of creatinine generation, and its volume of distribution. As a result, large changes in GFR may be associated with relatively small changes in SCr in the first 2448 hrs following CSA-AKI, resulting not only in delayed diagnosis and intervention but also in underestimation of the severity of CSA-AKI [63-65].

Biomarkers for AKI

Recently a variety genes or gene products have been identified which serve as biomarkers for AKI. These biomarkers are able to aid in early detection of AKI even before the rise in SCr. They have the potential to improve both the sensitivity and specificity of detecting ischemic CSA-AKI [66]. However, biomarkers are also needed for: (a) discerning CSA-AKI subtypes (prerenal, intrinsic renal, or postrenal), (b) identifying CSA-AKI etiologies (ischemia, toxins, sepsis, or a combination), severity and course of CSA-AKI, (c) differentiating CSA-AKI from other forms of AKI (glomerulonephritis, acute tubulointerstitial nephritis), (f) monitoring the response to interventions [67].

Biomarkers may detect CSA-AKI early in the tissue injury phase, several hours before the increase in SCr and provide a window of opportunity for effective therapies that may alter the clinical outcomes of CSA-AKI patients such as less severe CSA-AKI, decreased need for dialysis, reduced duration of CSA-AKI, improved short and long-term mortality and progression of chronic kidney disease [66]. Although, there have been more than 20 unique biomarkers of AKI identified or under investigation, most of the current interest has focused on a handful of promising biomarkers: NGAL, cystatin C, IL-18, and KIM-1 [68].

Neutrophil gelatinase–associated lipocalin (NGAL): In the setting of cardiac surgery, NGAL is a highly sensitive and specific biomarker of CSA-AKI [69-71]. Mishra et al. found that both urine and serum NGAL increased 2 hours after CPB and were found to be the most powerful independent predictors of AKI [69]. Dent et al. has demonstrated that both Ur-NGAL (at 2 hours) and plasma NGAL (at 12 hours) strongly correlate with mortality in children [70, 72]. Similar results have been observed in the adult cardiac surgical population [71]. In a study of 81 adult cardiac patients, where 20% of the patients developed CSA-AKI, NGAL was higher in patients with CSA-AKI at 1, 3 and 18 hours post-CPB [73].

Interleukin-18 (IL-18): IL-18 is an IL-1 subgroup proinflammatory cytokine, and is found to be a mediator and biomarker of ischemic AKI. Parikh et al. found that urine IL-18 was detectable at 4 to 6 hours, peaked at 12 hours, and remained elevated for more than 48 hours in patients with AKI [74].

Kidney injury molecule-1 (KIM-1): Study by Liangos et al. showed that KIM-1 levels increased significantly at both 2 and 24 hours postoperatively in patients with AKI [75].

Cystatin C: Few studies have explored cystatin C as a biomarker for CSA-AKI. Van De Voorde et al. found that both cystatin C and NGAL were very strong independent predictors of CSA-AKI [76] NGAL was elevated 2 hours postoperatively, whereas cystatin C was elevated at 12 hours postoperatively. Koyner et al., measured cystatin C and NGAL in serum and urine in post CPB adults. Within the first 6 hours, serum values for both cystatin C and NGAL were not predictive of AKI whereas urinary values were elevated [77]. These findings suggest that urinary biomarkers may be superior to serum values for early detection of CSA-AKI.

Diagnostic Issues with Biomarkers

Despite the promise for earlier AKI detection with greater sensitivity, almost all of them have certain limitations. NGAL is influenced by preexisting renal disease and infections [78,79]. KIM-1 is specific to ischemic and nephrotoxic causes of AKI only and not useful for other AKI subtypes [80,81]. IL-18 peaks later than many other leading biomarkers at 4-6 hours postoperatively and is more specific for ischemic AKI [74]. Finally, Cystatin C is not specific for ischemic AKI and increase occurs much later than NGAL, KIM-1, and IL-18 [76]. The role of widespread use of biomarkers for early detection of AKI remains questionable because of above mentioned drawbacks and lack of successful therapeutic interventions after early diagnosis. However, they are extremely valuable in research scenarios, specifically in clinical trials involving therapeutic interventions for AKI.

Prevention and Treatment of CSA-AKI

Bothe non-pharmacologic and pharmacological interventions have been proposed and investigated in prevention and treatment trials of AKI. Non-pharmacological interventions include close monitoring and adjustment of volume status, avoidance of nephrotoxins and modifications in surgical techniques such as off pump bypass or hypothermia. Since hemodynamic problems contribute significantly to the pathogenesis of CSA-AKI, hemodynamic management is of paramount importance [82]. The term "goal-directed therapy" is used to describe the use of cardiac output or similar parameters to guide intravenous fluid and inotropic therapy [83]. Different approaches including inotropic agents, fluids or both used to maximize oxygen delivery [84,85]. Studies about timing of such therapy (pre, intra or postoperatively) have generally been more positive [86, 87].

Pharmacological interventions have been attempted with inconsistent results, and so far there are no known drugs that have demonstrated renal protection. This may be related to the following factors: 1) the pathophysiology of CSA-AKI is complex, and simple approaches to target single pathways are unlikely to succeed; 2) late pharmacological intervention is likely to meet with failure; and 3) patients who were studied were often at low risk for renal dysfunction post-CPB, thus potentially masking small beneficial effects of therapies. Most therapeutic trials in CSA-AKI have been prevention studies in which treatment was initiated before the insult and, in the majority of cases, have shown no significant benefits [88].

Non-Pharmacologic Interventions in CSA-AKI

Non-pharmacologic strategies include preoperative fluid loading, avoiding the use of CPB and aortic manipulation, and preemptive RRT [82]. Treatment of volume depletion and CHF before cardiac surgery should target optimizing cardiac output and renal perfusion. There are no guidelines to choose a specific fluid or vasoactive drug to improve renal function [89,90]. Hydration is a universally accepted strategy to prevent contrast nephropathy; however, its use in the CSA-AKI has not been thoroughly investigated. One should weigh the value of preoperative hydration against the risk of highly positive fluid balances leading to pulmonary complications, excessive hemodilution and blood transfusion [89].

It is unknown whether intraoperative optimization of bypass flow, perfusion pressure, and oxygen delivery would mitigate the progression of CSA-AKI. Several trials have demonstrated a significant reduction in the incidence of CSA-AKI with off-pump surgery.

However, Cheng et al. could not confirm these findings in their study (91) although Sajja et al. showed in patients with preoperative CKD a beneficial effect on postoperative SCr and need for dialysis [92].

Avoidance of Nephrotoxins

It is known that there is a deleterious effect of aprotinin (Antifibrolytic) on postoperative kidney function [93], and use of radiocontrast agents within 48 hours before cardiac surgery is an independent risk factor for postoperative AKI. The use of ACE-inhibitors (ACEI) and Angiotensin Receptor Blockers (ARB) in the perioperative period of cardiac surgery remains controversial. Some recommend discontinuing these drugs the day before surgery [82]. Studies on the use of NSAID's for the treatment of postoperative pain don't show a significant deleterious effect on renal function in elective CABG patients [94] however, their use should generally be avoided in these situations specifically in patients with preexisting CKD.

Pharmacological Interventions in Preventing and Treating CSA-AKI

The efficacy of a number of pharmacological interventions has been evaluated in the prevention and management of AKI. These interventions can be separated into measures designed to improve renal perfusion and/or glomerular function, promote natriuresis and block inflammation [89].

1- Drugs That Increase Renal Blood Flow

Dopamine: At low doses, it stimulates DA-1 and DA-2 receptors, and thereby decreases renal vascular resistance and enhances diuresis and natriuresis. Although dopamine has been used extensively in these scenarios, studies have failed to show its efficacy in CSA-AKI [95]. The overall lack of efficacy of low-dose dopamine was reported in Friedrich et al. in their meta-analysis [96]. Another meta-analysis was done by Kellum et al. also found that dopamine failed to reduce the incidence of AKI, need for dialysis or risk of death [97]. However, there was concern for potential toxicity, including tachycardia, arrhythmias, myocardial ischemia, and intestinal ischemia. Thus dopamine cannot be recommended as a renal protective agent and better be avoided.

Fenoldopam: Fenoldopam is a selective DA-1 agonist that has been used for the prevention of AKI in small trials with variable results. Small studies using fenoldopam have demonstrated a reduction of renal dysfunction. However, Bove et al., found that in CKD patients undergoing cardiac surgery fenoldopam did not reduce the rate of CSA-AKI or need for dialysis [98]. Brienza et al. in study on AKI patients found that fenoldopam decreased SCr by 10%. However, the mean peak Cr and urine output did not change [99]. A potential complication of fenoldopam was systemic hypotension. The beneficial effect of renal vasodilatation in this situation may be offset by systemic hypotension and therefore should be avoided.

Theophylline: It is thought to block vasoconstriction induced by A1-AR and thus increase renal blood flow. However, it was found that theophylline infusion in coronary bypass surgery was ineffective in reducing the incidence of AKI [100].

2. Drugs That Induce Natriuresis

Natriuretic Peptides (ANP and BNP)

ANP: They increase GFR due to arteriolar dilatation and also have a natriuretic effect by inhibiting sodium reabsorption by the medullary collecting duct. Sward et al. found that use of ANP was associated with a significant reduction in the incidence of dialysis at day 21 of CSA-AKI [101]. Bergman et al. and Sezai et al. showed a beneficial effect of ANP on kidney function [102,103]. However, a trial by Hayashida et al. did not find any beneficial effect on kidney function with use of ANP intraoperatively during cardiac surgery [104]. The potential benefit of vasodilatation may have been negated by the presence of hypotension.

Nesiritide (BNP): Beaver et al. found reduced risk of dialysis or death in patients with SCr > 1.0mg/dL; however, no effect was noted in patients with preoperative SCr < 1.0mg/dL [105]. Ejaz et al., in their randomized controlled trial showed no benefit of prophylactic nesiritide on the incidence of RRT and/or death in high risk cardiac surgery [106]. Mentzer at al demonstrated favorable short-term effects on renal function however larger randomized controlled trials are required to further evaluate its role in prevention of CSA-AKI [107].

Diuretics: theoretically they may reduce the severity of CSA-AKI by preventing tubule obstruction and decrease O2 consumption by inhibition of the Na-K-2Cl co-transporter. Diuretics are commonly used to enhance urine output, convert oliguria to non-oliguria, or maintain urine output in setting of large infusions of fluid. Studies of diuretics for the prevention or reversal of CSA-AKI have shown inconsistent results; Lassnigg et al. found that furosemide was not protective as the incidence of CSA-AKI was twice that of the dopamine or placebo group [108]. Mehta et al. found that diuretics increased the risk of death and nonrecovery of renal function [109]. In a study done by Sirivella et al. in oliguric CSA-AKI a cocktail infusion of furosemide, mannitol and dopamine improved renal function compared to intermittent loop diuretics alone [110]. However, numerous studies in patients with established AKI have found no benefit of loop diuretics. Thus, the routine use of diuretics may not be warranted and should be avoided.

Mannitol: It may help to maintain urine output during the procedure, minimize tissue edema, and serve as a free-radical scavenger; the potential role of mannitol remains unclear. Ip-Yam et al. showed that the use of prophylactic mannitol did not produce any significant differences in Ur-microalbumin, Ur-NAG, FeNa, and SCr. [111]. Carcoana et al. showed an increased urinary excretion of 2-microglobulin in patients receiving mannitol and dopamine, suggestive of increased tubular injury [112].

3-Drugs That Block Inflammation

Inflammatory mediators are attractive therapeutic targets for the prevention of CSA-AKI.

Pentoxifylline: a phosphodiesterase inhibitor, blocks the activation of neutrophils by TNF-alfa and IL-1 and TNF-alfa release by inflammatory cells. It reduces cardiac dysfunction and TNF-alfa release in ischemia-reperfusion models. However, it was not found to affect renal function in patients undergoing cardiac surgery [113].

Dexamethasone: Study done with dexamethasone failed to show any protection against CSA-AKI. [114]

N-acetylcysteine (N-AC): a thiol-containing antioxidant, has been investigated primarily for the prevention of contrast – induced nephropathy with inconclusive results. Burns et al. studied N-AC for the prevention of CSA-AKI and found no significant difference in any outcome with its use [115]. A small study done by Fisher et al. suggested that N-AC protects kidney function in patients undergoing CBP [116], however, Haase et al. conducted a phase II clinical trial and found that N-AC was no more effective than placebo in attenuating CSA-AKI [117]. In conclusion existing evidence does not support the use of NAC to prevent CSA-AKI.

4. Other Pharmacological Strategies:

Clonidine (an alpha-2 agonist): The sympathetic nervous system is activated during cardiac surgery and may lead to impairment of renal function through a hemodynamic mechanism. Clonidine has been used to attenuate these effects, with improvement in hemodynamic stability during CPB. Kulka et al. found that preoperative treatment with clonidine prevented the deterioration of renal function [118], however other trials have shown inconsistent results.

Diltiazem: has been shown to inhibit some inflammatory effects of CPB and is often used to prevent vasospasm of radial grafts. Although diltiazem reduces Urinary markers of tubule injury, its effectiveness in the prevention of CSA-AKI was inconsistent and its use cannot be recommended [119,120].

Various other therapeutic agents such as growth factors and erythropoietin have shown promise in the early stages of investigation and need further evaluation.

Treatment of Established CSA-AKI (Extracorporeal Therapy, RRT)

Several studies have evaluated the timing for initiation, mode and intensity of extracorporeal therapy for CSA-AKI. Some studies have demonstrated potential survival benefit with earlier initiation and continuous therapy. However, to date studies remain inconsistent about any advantage with particular method of RRT or timing of initiation [89].

Generally, it is preferred to initiate RRT for uremic symptoms or signs, or for refractory volume overload, electrolyte abnormalities or acidosis. Initiation of RRT in patients with progressive azotemia prior to the development of overt uremic manifestations is associated with better survival; some studies suggest that more intensive delivery of renal support during AKI is associated with improved survival [121,122].

Mode of RRT (Intermittent Hemodialysis (IHD) vs. Continuous Renal Replacement Therapy (CRRT))

Conventional IHD is associated with higher hemodynamic instability than CRRT, and therefore CRRT is considered the safer modality for treatment of CSA- AKI in the critical care setup. This is because IHD is more likely to cause hypotensive episodes which are highly undesirable for the AKI recovery [124]. CRRT also allows a greater metabolic control to be achieved and thus provides a platform for an aggressive, protein rich nutritional policy to improve daily nitrogen balance, thus having possible favorable effects on immune function and overall outcome [125]. CRRT helps decrease myocardial edema, reduce left ventricular end diastolic pressure by optimizing the Frank-Starling relationship and improving myocardial performance by removing circulating myocardial depressants [126,127].

Various forms of CRRT are available to use in CSA-AKI (Continuous veno-venous hemofiltration-CVVH, Continuous veno-venous hemodialysis-CVVHD, Continuous veno-venous hemodiafiltration-CVVHDF, and Continuous arterio-venous hemodialysis-CAVHD). Application of specific type of continuous renal replacement therapy (CRRT) is usually tailored to the patient's need (patient characteristics, urgency of treatment, hemodynamic tolerance and vascular access). In addition, nutrition should be considered as an integral part of all RRT prescription taking into account the degree of catabolism [123]. Although CRRT appears to have certain advantages over IHD, randomized controlled studies have failed to show any consistent benefits in terms of short term or long term mortality with CRRT over IHD.

Alternate Day IHD versus Daily IHD

Schiffl et al. reported the effect of daily IHD, as compared with conventional (alternate-day) IHD, on survival among patients with AKI. They concluded that daily HD resulted in better control of uremia, fewer hypotensive episodes during HD, and more rapid resolution of AKI than did conventional HD. The mortality rate was 28% for daily HD and 46% for alternate-day HD, and it was found that alternate day HD was an independent risk factor for death [128].

Timing of Initiation (Early versus Late)

Bouman et al. studied the effects of the initiation time of CVVH and ultrafiltration (UF) and of the UF rate and found that survival at 28 days and recovery of renal function were not improved using high ultrafiltrate volumes or early initiation [129]. Bent et al. and Elahi et al. based on their study concluded that early and aggressive use of CVVH is associated with better survival in CSA-AKI [130,131].

Effect of Duration and Intensity of CRRT

Several studies have failed to demonstrate outcome improvement with more intense RRT; Palevsky et al. suggest that the duration of intense versus less-intense RRT did not affect the outcomes [132]. Paganini et al. found that the larger dialysis delivery dose is associated with better outcomes [125]. Tolwani et al. studied the effect of dosage of CVVHDF on survival in patients with ARF, a significant difference in patient survival or renal recovery was not detected between patients receiving high-dosage or standard-dosage CVVHDF [133].

Elimination of Inflammatory Cytokines and Anaphylatoxins by CRRT

CRRT may also help in removing inflammatory mediators like TNF alpha and cytokines. However, most of these mediators are larger in size and may not freely pass through the filters. Existing data is inconclusive about removal of TNF alpha or other inflammatory mediators by CRRT [123].

Ongoing Trials

Erythropoietin has been shown to have diverse effects on nonhematopoeitic tissues that may be beneficial in the prevention of AKI. One such effect is the direct action of erythropoietin on polymorphonuclear leukocytes to decrease systemic inflammation and oxidative stress [134]. Another promising treatment for the prevention of AKI is minocycline (via its anti-inflammatory and antiapoptotic properties) [135]. Elahi et al. are currently conducting a study to evaluate its efficacy preoperatively in CKD patients undergoing cardiac surgery [136].

Intrarenal infusion of medications is another emerging therapy proposed to improve efficacy and decrease the systemic effects of renal protective therapies. Intrarenal fenoldopam has been used successfully in several case reports and a small pilot trial, but there is not enough data in CSA-AKI population [137,138].

Conclusion

Therapeutic interventions in cardiac surgery have not produced consistent favorable results due to lack of understanding of the mechanisms of CSA-AKI, non-uniformity of study designs, heterogeneity of study population, lack of uniform definition, drug dosage and durations and absence of reliable early biomarkers of renal injury. However, there has been tremendous stride in all aspects of this serious complication of cardiac surgery. These advances in pathomechanisms, diagnosis and treatment need to be validated in large clinical studies before they can be introduced into routine clinical practice. Prevention by rigorous preoperative risk stratification, decreasing intraoperative risk variables and management of postoperative traditional and non-traditional risk factors may be more important than the treatment of established CSA-AKI.

References

[1]   Conlon PJ, Stafford-Smith M, White WD, et al. Acute renal failure following cardiac surgery. *Nephrol Dial Transplant* 1999;14:1158–1162. [PubMed: 10344355].

[2]   Abraham VS, Swain JA. Cardiopulmonary bypass and the kidney. In: *Cardiopulmonary Bypass: Principles and Practice,* 2nd Ed., edited by Gravlee GP, Davis RF, Kurusz M, Utley JR, Philadelphia, Lippincott Williams & Wilkins, 2000, pp 382–391.

[3] Grayson AD, et al: Valvular heart operation is an independent risk factor for acute renal failure. *Ann Thorac Surg* 75: 1829–1835, 2003.

[4] Mangano CM, et al: Renal dysfunction after myocardial revascularization: Risk factors, adverse outcomes and hospital resource utilization. *Ann Intern Med* 128: 194– 203, 1998.

[5] Abel RM, et al: Etiology, incidence and prognosis of renal failure following cardiac operations. Results of a prospective analysis of 500 consecutive patients. *J Thorac Cardiovasc Surg* 71: 323–333, 1976.

[6] Gailiunas P Jr, et al: Acute renal failure following cardiac operations. *J Thorac Cardiovasc Surg* 79: 241–243, 1980.

[7] Ostermann ME, et al: Acute renal failure following cardiopulmonary bypass: A changing picture. *Intensive Care Med* 26: 565–571, 2000.

[8] Mangos GJ, et al: Acute renal failure following cardiac surgery: Incidence, outcomes and risk factors. *Aust N Z J Med* 25: 284–289, 1995.

[9] Antunes PE, et al: Renal dysfunction alter myocardial revascularization. *Eur J Cardiothorac Surg* 25: 597–604, 2004.

[10] Yeboah ED, et al: Acute renal failure and open heart surgery. *BMJ* 1: 415–418, 1972.

[11] Bhat JG, et al: Renal failure after open heart surgery. *Ann Intern Med* 84: 677–682, 1976.

[12] Hilberman M, et al: Acute renal failure following cardiac surgery. *J Thorac Cardiovasc Surg* 77: 880–888, 1979.

[13] Corwin HL, et al: Acute renal failure associated with cardiac operations. A casecontrol study. *J Thorac Cardiovasc Surg* 98: 1107–1112, 1989.

[14] Schmitt H, et al: Acute renal failure following cardiac surgery: Pre- and perioperative clinical features. *Contrib Nephrol* 93: 98–104, 1991.

[15] Chertow GM, et al: Independent association between acute renal failure and mortality following cardiac surgery. *Am J Med* 104: 343–348, 1998.

[16] Lassnigg A, et al: Minimal changes of serum creatinine predict prognosis in patients after cardiothoracic surgery: A prospective cohort study. *J Am Soc Nephrol* 15: 1597–1605, 2004.

[17] Thakar CV, et al: Influence of renal dysfunction on mortality after cardiac surgery: Modifying effect of preoperative renal function. *Kidney Int* 67: 1112–1119, 2005.

[18] Dasta et al, Costs and outcomes of acute kidney injury (AKI) following cardiac Surgery *Nephrol Dial Transplant* (2008) 23: 1970–1974.

[19] Chertow GM, Lazarus JM, Christiansen CL, et al. Preoperative renal risk stratification. *Circulation* 1997;95:878–884. [PubMed: 9054745].

[20] Thakar CV, et al. A clinical score to predict acute renal failure after cardiac surgery. *J Am Soc Nephrol* 2005;16:162–168. [PubMed: 15563569].

[21] Wijeysundera DN, et al. Derivation and validation of a simplified predictive index for renal replacement therapy after cardiac surgery. *JAMA* 2007;297:1801–1809.[PubMed: 17456822].

[22] Palomba H, et al. Acute kidney injury prediction following elective cardiac surgery: AKICS score. *Kidney Int* 2007;72:624–631. [PubMed: 17622275].

[23] Fortescue EB, et al: Predicting acute Clin J Am Soc Nephrol 1: 19–32, 2006 Cardiac Surgery and Acute Kidney Injury renal failure after coronary bypass surgery: Cross-validation of two risk-stratification algorithms. *Kidney Int* 57: 2594–2602, 2000.

[24] Frost L, et al: Prognosis and risk factors in acute, dialysis-requiring renal failure after open-heart surgery. *Scand J Thorac Cardiovasc Surg* 25: 161–166, 1991.

[25] Thakar CV, et al: ARF after open-heart surgery: Influence of gender and race. *Am J Kidney Dis* 41: 742–751, 2003.

[26] Thakar CV, Liangos O, Yared J-P, Nelson DA, Hariachar S, Paganini EP: Predicting acute renal failure after cardiac surgery: Validation and re-definition of a risk stratification algorithm. *Hemodial Int* 7: 143–147, 2003.

[27] Slogoff S, et al.: Role of perfusion pressure and flow in major organ dysfunction after cardiopulmonary bypass. *Ann Thorac Surg* 50: 911–918, 1990.

[28] Tuttle KR, et al: Predictors of ARF after cardiac surgical procedures. *Am J Kidney Dis* 41: 76–83, 2003.

[29] Fischer UM, et al: Impact of cardiopulmonary bypass management on postcardiac surgery renal function. *Perfusion* 17: 401–406, 2002.

[30] Abramov D, et al: The influence of cardiopulmonary bypass flow characteristics on the clinical outcome of 1820 coronary bypass patients. *Can J Cardiol* 19: 237–243, 2003.

[31] Urzua J, et al. Renal function and cardiopulmonary bypass: Effect of perfusion pressure. *J Cardiothorac Vasc Anesth* 6: 299–303, 1992.

[32] Provenchere S, et al. : Renal dysfunction after cardiac surgery with normothermic cardiopulmonary bypass: Incidence, risk factors and effect on clinical outcome. *Anesth Analg* 96: 1258–1264, 2003.

[33] The Warm Heart Investigators: Randomized trial of normothermic versus hypothermic coronary artery bypass surgery. *Lancet* 343: 559–563, 1994.

[34] Cook DJ: Changing temperature management for cardiopulmonary bypass. *Anesth Analg* 88: 1254–1271, 1999.

[35] Magee MJ, Edgerton JR: Beating heart coronary artery bypass: Operative strategy and technique. *Sem Thorac Cardiovasc Surg* 15: 83–91, 2003.

[36] Loef BG, et al: Off-pump coronary revascularization attenuates transient renal damage compared with on-pump coronary revascularization. *Chest* 121: 1190–1194, 2002.

[37] Ascione R, et al: On-pump versus off-pump coronary revascularization: Evaluation of renal function. *Ann Thorac Surg* 68: 493–498, 1999.

[38] Schwann NM, et al: Does off-pump coronary artery bypass reduce the incidence of clinically evident renal dysfunction after multivessel myocardial revascularization? *Anesth Analg* 99: 959–964, 2004.

[39] Beauford RB, et al: Is off-pump revascularization better for patients with non-dialysis-dependent renal insufficiency? *Heart Surg Forum* 7: E141–146, 2004.

[40] Gamboso MG, et al: Off-pump versus on-pump coronary artery bypass surgery and post-operative renal dysfunction. *Anesth Analg* 91: 1080–1084, 2000.

[41] Stallwood MI, et al: Acute renal failure in coronary artery bypass surgery: Independent effect of cardiopulmonary bypass. *Ann Thorac Surg* 77: 968–972, 2004.

[42] Hudson et al. Emerging Concepts in Acute Kidney Injury Following Cardiac Surgery *Semin Cardiothorac Vasc Anesth.* 2008 December; 12(4): 320–330. doi:10.1177/1089253208328582.

[43] Mitchell et al, Acute Kidney Injury Associated with Cardiac Surgery *Clin J Am Soc Nephrol* 1: 19–32, 2006.

[44] Finn A, Naik S, Klein N, Levinsky RJ, Strobel S, Elliott M. Interleukin-8 release and neutrophil degranulation after pediatric cardiopulmonary bypass. *J Thorac Cardiovasc Surg* 1993; 105: 234–41.

[45] Bellomo et al, The pathophysiology of cardiac surgery-associated acute kidney injury (CSA-AKI) *The International Journal of Artificial Organs* / Vol. 31 / no. 2, 2008 / pp. 166-178.

[46] Wright G: Hemolysis during cardiopulmonary bypass: Update. *Perfusion* 16: 345–351, 2001.

[47] Fransen E, et al. W: Systemic inflammation present in patients undergoing CABG without extracorporeal circulation. *Chest* 113: 1290–1295, 1998.

[48] Dybdahl B, Wahba A, Haaverstad R, Kirkeby-Garstad I, Kierulf P, Espevik T, Sundan A: On-pump versus offpump coronary artery bypass grafting: More heat-shock protein 70 is released after on-pump surgery. *Eur J Cardiothorac Surg* 25: 985–992, 2004.

[49] Sheridan AM, Bonventre JV: Cell biology and molecular mechanisms of injury in ischemic acute renal failure. *Curr Opin Nephrol Hypertens* 9: 427–434, 2000.

[50] Molitoris BA: Transitioning to therapy in ischemic acute renal failure. *J Am Soc Nephrol* 14: 265–267, 2003.

[51] Sutton TA, et al: Microvascular endothelial injury and dysfunction during ischemic acute renal failure. *Kidney Int* 62: 1539–1549, 2002.

[52] Conger JD: Vascular alterations in acute renal failure: Roles in initiation and maintenance. In: *Acute Renal Failure—A Companion to Brenner and Rector's The Kidney,* edited by Molitoris BA, Finn WF, Philadelphia, Saunders, 2001, pp13–29.

[53] Okusa MD: The inflammatory cascade in acute ischemic renal failure *Nephron* 90: 133–138, 2002.

[54] Shinji Hirai , Systemic Inflammatory Response Syndrome after Cardiac Surgery under *Cardiopulmonary Bypass Ann Thorac Cardiovasc Surg* Vol. 9, No. 6 365-370 (2003).

[55] Hornick P, Taylor KM: Immune and inflammatory responses after cardiopulmonary bypass. In: *Cardiopulmonary Bypass: Principles and Practice*, edited by Gravlee GP, Davis RF, Kurusz M, Utley JR, Philadelphia, Lippincott Williams & Wilkins, 2000, pp 303–320.

[56] Asimakopoulos G, Taylor KM: Effects of cardiopulmonary bypass on leukocyte and endothelial adhesion molecules. *Ann Thorac Surg* 66: 2135–2144, 1998.

[57] Galinanes M, et al: Differential patterns of neutrophil adhesion molecules during cardiopulmonary bypass in humans. *Circulation* 94[Suppl 2]: 364–369, 1996.

[58] Zilla P, et al: Blood platelets in cardiopulmonary bypass operations. *J Thorac Cardiovasc Surg* 97: 379–388, 1989.

[59] Gutteridge JMC: Iron promoters of the Fenton reaction and lipid peroxidation can be released from hemoglobin by peroxides. *Fed Eur Biochem Soc Lett* 201: 291–295, 1986.

[60] Flaherty JT, Weisfeldt ML: Reperfusion injury. *Free Radic Biol Med* 5: 409–419, 1988

[61] Laffey JG, Boylan JF, Cheng DC. The systemic inflammatory response to cardiac surgery: implications for the anesthesiologist. *Anesthesiology* 2002;97:215–252.

[62] Vaidya VS1, Ozer JS, Frank D, Collings FB, Ramirez V, Troth S, Muniappa N, Thudium D, Gerhold D,Holder DJ, Bobadilla NA, Marrer E, Perentes E, Cordier A, Vonderscher J, Maurer G, Goering PL, Sistare FD, and Bonventre JV et al. Nat Biotechnol. Kidney Injury Molecule-1 Outperforms Traditional Biomarkers of Kidney

Injury in Multi-site Preclinical Biomarker Qualification Studies2010 May ; 28(5): 478–485.

[63] Bellomo R, Ronco C, Kellum JA, et al., Acute Dialysis Quality Initiative workgroup. Acute renal failure—definition, outcome measures, animal models, fluid therapy, and information tech- nology needs: The Second International Consensus Conference of the Acute Dialysis Quality Initiative (ADQI) *Group. Crit Care* 2004;8:R204.

[64] Arnaoutakis GJ, Bihorac A, Martin TD, et al. RIFLE criteria for acute kidney injury in aortic arch surgery. *J Thorac Cardiovasc Surg* 2007;134:1554.

[65] Vaidya VS, Ferguson MA, Bonventre JVet al. Biomarkers of acute kidney injury, *The Annual Review of Pharmacology and Toxicology* 2008 ; 48: 463–493.

[66] Hudson C, Hudson J, Swaminathan M, Shaw A , Stafford-Smith M, Patel UD et al. Emerging concepts in acute kidney injury following cardiac surgery. *Semin Cardiothorac Vasc Anesth.* 2008 December ; 12(4): 320–330.

[67] Nguyen MT , Devarajan P et al, Biomarkers for the early detection of acute kidney injury, *Pediatr Nephrol* (2008) 23:2151–2157.

[68] Edelstein CL. Biomarkers of acute kidney injury. *Adv Chronic Kidney Dis* 2008; 15:222-234.

[69] Mishra J, Dent C, Tarabishi R, et al. Neutrophil gelatinase-associated lipocalin (NGAL) as a biomarker for acute renal injury after cardiac surgery. *Lancet* 2005;365:1231–1238.

[70] Dent CL, Ma Q, Dastrala S, et al. Plasma neutrophil gelatinase-associated lipocalin predicts acute kidney injury, morbidity and mortality after pediatric cardiac surgery: a prospective uncontrolled cohort study. *Crit Care* 2007;11:R127.

[71] Wagener G, Jan M, Kim M, et al. Association between increases in urinary neutrophil gelatinase- associated lipocalin and acute renal dysfunction after adult cardiac surgery. *Anesthesiology* 2006;105:485–491.

[72] Bennett M, Dent CL, Ma Q, et al. Urine NGAL predicts severity of acute kidney injury after cardiac surgery: a prospective study. *Clin J Am Soc Nephrol* 2008;3:665–673.

[73] Wagener G, Gubitosa G, Wang S, Borregaard N, Kim M, Lee HT. Increased incidence of acute kidney injury with aprotinin use during cardiac surgery detected with urinary NGAL. *Am J Nephrol* 2008;28:576–582.

[74] Parikh CR, Mishra J, Thiessen-Philbrook H, et al. Urinary IL-18 is an early predictive biomarker of acute kidney injury after cardiac surgery. *Kidney Int* 2006;70:199–203.

[75] Liangos O, Han WK, Wald R, et al. Urinary kidney injury molecule-1 level is an early and sensitive marker of acute kidney injury. *J Am Soc Nephrol* 2006; 17:403A.

[76] Van de Voorde RG, Katlman TI, Ma Q, et al. Serum NGAL and cystatin C as predictive biomarkers for acute kidney injury . *J Am Soc Nephrol* 2006;17:404A.

[77] Koyner JL, Bennett MR, Worcester EM, et al. Urinary cystatin C as an early biomarker of acute kidney injury following adult cardiothoracic surgery. *Kidney Int* 2008;74:1059–1069.

[78] Mitsnefes MM, Kathman TS, Mishra J, et al. Serum neutrophil gelatinase-associated lipocalin as a marker of renal function in children with chronic kidney disease. *Pediatr Nephrol* 2007;22:101– 108.

[79] Pisitkun T, Johnstone R, Knepper MA. Discovery of urinary biomarkers. *Mol Cell Proteomics* 2006;5:1760–1771.

[80] Han WK, Bailly V, Abichandani R, Thadhani R, Bonventre JV. Kidney Injury Molecule-1 (KIM-1): a novel biomarker for human renal proximal tubule injury. *Kidney Int* 2002;62:237–244.

[81] Han WK, Waikar SS, Johnson A, Curhan GC, Devarajan P, Bonventre JV. Urinary biomarkers for early detection of acute kidney injury . *J Am Soc Nephrol* 2006;17:403A.

[82] Schetz M, Bove T., Morelli A, Mankad S. , Ronco , Kellum JA. Prevention of cardiac surgery-associated acute kidney injury. *The International Journal of Artificial Organs* / Vol. 31 / no. 2, 2008 / pp. 179-189.

[83] Pearse R, Dawson D, Fawcett J, Rhodes A, Grounds RM, Bennett ED. Early goal directed therapy after major surgery reduces complications and duration of hospital stay. A rando- mised, controlled trial. *Crit Care* 2005; 9: R687-93.

[84] Kern JW, Shoemaker WC. Meta-analysis of hemodynamic optimisation in high risk patients. *Crit Care Med* 2002; 30: 1686-92.

[85] PoezeM,GreveJW,RamsayG.Meta-analysisofhemodyna- mic optimisation: relationship to methodological quality. *Crit Care* 2005; 9: R771-9.

[86] BoydO,GroundsRM,BennetED.Arandomizedclinicaltrial on the effect of deliberate perioperative increase of oxygen delivery on mortality in high risk surgical patients. *JAMA* 1993; 270: 2699-707.

[87] WilsonJ,WoodsI,FawcettJ,WhallR,DibbW,MorrisC,Mc- Manus E. Reducing the risk of major elective surgery: rando- mized controlled trial of preoperative optimisation of oxygen delivery. *BMJ* 1999; 318: 1099-1103.

[88] Rosner MH, Portilla D, Okusa MD. Cardiac surgery as a cause of acute kidney injury: Pathogenesis and Potential Therapies. *J Intensive Care Med.* 2008 Jan-Feb;23(1):3-18.

[89] Tolwani A, Paganini E, Joannisis M, Zamperetti N, Verbine A, Vidyasagar V, Clark W, Ronco C et al. Treatment odf patients with cardiac surgery associated- acute kidney injury. *The International Journal of Artificial Organs* / Vol. 31 / no. 2, 2008 / pp. 190-196.

[90] Roberts I, Alderson P, Bunn F, Chinnock, P, Ker K, Schierhout G. Colloids versus crystalloids for fluid resuscitation in criti- cally ill patients Cochrane Database of Systematic Reviews 2007 Issue 2. Roberts I, Alderson P, Bunn F, Chinnock, P, Ker K, Schierhout G. Colloids versus crystalloids for fluid resuscitation in criti- cally ill patients *Cochrane Database of Systematic Reviews* 2007 Issue 2.

[91] Cheng DC, Bainbridge D, Martin JE, Novick RJ; Evidence- Based Perioperative Clinical Outcomes Research Group. Does off-pump coronary artery bypass reduce mortality, mor- bidity, and resource utilization when compared with conven- tional coronary artery bypass? A meta-analysis of randomi- zed trials. *Anesthesiology* 2005; 102: 188-203.

[92] Sajja LR, Mannam G, Chakravarthi RM, Sompalli S, Naidu SK, Somaraju B, Penumatsa RR. Coronary artery bypass grafting with or without cardiopulmonary bypass in patients with preoperative non-dialysis dependent renal insufficiency: a randomized study. *J Thorac Cardiovasc Surg* 2007; 133: 378-88.

[93] Mangano DT, Tudor IC, Dietzel C; Multicenter Study of Perio- perative Ischemia Research Group; Ischemia Research and Education Foundation. The risk associated with aprotinin in cardiac surgery. *N Engl J Med* 2006; 354: 353-65.

[94] Hynninen MS, Cheng DC, Hossain I, Carroll J, Aumbhagavan SS, Yue R, Karski JM. Non-steroidal anti-inflammatory drugs in treatment of postoperative pain after cardiac surgery. *Can J Anesth* 2000; 47: 1182-7.

[95] Rosner MH, Portilla D, Okusa MD., Cardiac surgery as a cause of acute kidney injury: pathogenesis and potential therapies. *J Intensive Care ed.* 2008 Jan-Feb;23(1):3-18.

[96] Friedrich JO, Adhikari N, Herridge MS, Beyene J. Meta-analysis: low-dose dopamine increases urine out- put but does not prevent renal dysfunction or death. *Ann Intern Med.* 2005;142:510-520.

[97] Kellum J, Decker J. Use of dopamine in acute renal failure: A me- ta-analysis. *Crit Care Med* 2001; 29: 1526-31.

[98] Bove T, Landoni G, Calabro MG, et al. Renoprotective action of fenoldopam in high-risk patients undergoing cardiac surgery: a prospective, double-blind, random- ized clinical trial. *Circulation.* 2005;111:3230-3236.

[99] Brienza N, Malcangi V, Dalfino L, et al. A comparison between fenoldopam and low-dose dopamine in early renal dysfunction of critically ill patients. *Crit Care Med.* 2006; 34:707-714.

[100] Kramer BK, Preuner J, Ebenburger A, et al. Lack of renoprotective effect of theophylline during aortocoro- nary bypass surgery. *Nephrol Dial Transplant.* 2002; 17:910-915.

[101] Sward K, Valsson F, Odencrants P, et al. Recombinant human atrial natriuretic peptide in ischemic acute renal failure: a randomized placebo controlled trial. *Crit Care Med.* 2004;32: 1310-1315.

[102] Bergman A, Odar-Cederlof I, Westman L,Ohqvist G. Effect of human atrial natriuretic peptide in patients after coronary ar- tery bypass surgery. *J Cardiothorac Vasc Anesth* 1996; 10: 490-5.

[103] Sezai A, Shiono M, Hata M, Iida M, Wakui S, Soeda M, Negi- shi N, Kasamaki Y, Saito S, Kato J, Sezai Y. Efficacy of conti- nous low-dose human atrial natriuretic peptide given from the beginning of cardiopulmonary bypass for thoracic aortic sur- gery. *Surg Today* 2006; 36: 508-14.

[104] Hayashida N, Chihara S, Kashikie H, Tayama E, Yokose S, Akasu K, Aoyagi S. Effects of intraoperative administration of atrial natriuretic peptide. *Ann Thorac Surg* 2000; 70: 1319-26.

[105] Beaver TM, Winterstein AG, Shuster JJ, Gerhard T, Martin T Alexander JA, Johnson RJ, Ejaz A, Hartzema AG. Effective- ness of nesiritide on dialysis or all.cause mortality in patients undergoing cardiothoracic surgery. *Clin Cardiol* 2006; 29: 18-24.

[106] Ejaz AA, Martin TD, Johnson RJ, Winterstein AG, Klodell CT, Hess PJ Jr, Ali AK, Whidden EM, Staples NL, Alexander JA, House-Fancher MA, Beaver TM. Prophylactic nesiritide does not prevent dialysis or all-cause mortality in patients undergoing high-risk cardiac surgery. *J Thorac Cardiovasc Surg.* 2009 Oct;138(4):959-64. Epub 2009 Jul 3.

[107] Mentzer RM, Oz Mc Sladen RN, et al. Effects of perioperative nesiritide in patients with left ventricular dysfunction under- going cardiac surgery. The NAPA Trial. *J Am Coll Cardiol* 2007; 49: 716-26.

[108] Lassnigg A, Donner E, Grubhofer G, et al. Lack of renoprotective effects of dopamine and furose- mide during cardiac surgery. *J Am Soc Nephrol.* 2000;11: 97-104.

[109] Mehta RL, Pascual MT, Soroko S, Chertow GM. Diuretics, mortality and nonrecovery of renal function in acute renal failure. *JAMA*. 2002;288:2547-2552.

[110] Sirivella A, Gielchinsky I, Parsonnet V. Mannitol, furosemide, and dopamine infusion in postoperative renal failure compli- cating cardiac surgery. *Ann Thorac Surg* 2000; 69: 501-6.

[111] Ip-YamPC,MurphyS,BainesM,FoxMA,DesmondMJ,In- nes PA. Renal function and proteinuria after cardiopulmonary bypass: the effects of temperature and mannitol. *Anesth Analg* 1994; 78: 842-7.

[112] Carcoana OV, Mathew JP, Davis E, et al. Mannitol and dopamine in patients undergoing cardiopulmonary bypass: a randomized clinical trial. *Anesth Analg.* 2003; 97:1222-1229.

[113] Boldt J, Brosch C, Piper SN, Suttner S, Lehmann A, Werling C. Influence of prophylactic use of pentoxi- fylline on postoperative organ function in elderly cardiac surgery patients. *Crit Care Med.* 2001;29: 952-958.

[114] Loef BG, Henning RH, Epema AH, et al. Effect of dexamethasone on perioperative renal function impair- ment during cardiac surgery with cardiopulmonary bypass. *Br J Anaesth.* 2004;93:793-798.

[115] Burns KE, Chu MW, Novick RJ, Fox SA, Gallo K, Martin CM, Stitt LW, Heidenheim AP, Myers ML, Moist L. Perioperative N- acetylcysteine to prevent renal dysfunction in high-risk pa- tients undergoing CABG surgery. *JAMA* 2005; 294: 342-50.

[116] Fisher UM, Tossios P, Mehlhorn U. Renal protection by radi- cal scavenging in cardiac surgery patients. *Curr Med Res Opin* 2005; 21: 1161-4.

[117] Haase M, Haase-Fielitz A, Bagshaw SM, Reade MC, Morgera S, Seevenayagam S, Matalanis G, Buxton B, Doolan L, Bello- mo R. Phase II, randomized, controlled trial of high-dose N- acetylcysteine in high-risk cardiac surgery patients. *Crit Care Med* 2007; 35: 1-8.

[118] Kulka PJ, Tryba M, Zenz M. Preoperative alpha2- adrenergic receptor agonists prevent the deterioration of renal function after cardiac surgery: results of a ran- domized, controlled trial. *Crit Care Med.* 1996;24: 947-952.

[119] Young EW, Diab A, Kirsh MM. Intravenous diltiazem and acute renal failure after cardiac operations. *Ann Thorac Surg.* 1998;65:1316-1319.

[120] Amar D, Fleisher M. Diltiazem treatment does not alter renal function after thoracic surgery. *Chest.* 2001;119: 1476-1479.

[121] Palevsky P. Clinical review: Timing and dose of continuous renal replacement therapy in acute kidney injury. *Crit Care* 2007; 11: 232.

[122] D'Intini V, Ronco C, Bonello M, Bellomo R. Renal replacement therapy in acute renal failure. Best Pract *Res Clin Anaesthe- siol* 2004; 18: 145-57.

[123] Elahi MA, Sanjay AA, Axel PB, Nadey HC, Bashir MD. Acute kidney injury following cardiac surgery: impact of early versus late haemofiltration on morbidity and mortality; *European Journal of Cardio-thoracic Surgery* 35 (2009) 854-863

[124] Conger JD. Does hemodialysis delay recovery from ARF? *Semin Dial* 1990;3:146-8.

[125] Paganini EP, Tapolay M, Goormastic M, Halstenberg W, Kozlowski L, Leblanc M, Lee JC, Moreno L, Sakai K. Establishing a dialysis therapy/ patient outcome link in intensive care unit acute dialysis for patients with acute renal failure. *Am J Kidney Dis* 1996;28:81-9.

[126] Cipolla CM, Grazi S, Rimondini A, Susini G, Guazzi M, Della Bella P, Guazzi MD. Changes in circulating norepinephrine with hemofiltration in advanced congestive heart failure. *Am J Cardiol* 1990 15;66:987-94.

[127] Caprioli R, Favilla G, Palmarini D, Comite C, Gemignani R, Rindi P, Cioni L. Automatic continuous venovenous hemodialfiltration in cardiosurgical patients. *ASAIO J* 1993;39:606-8.

[128] Schiffl H, Lang SM, Fischer R. Daily hemodialysis and the outcome of acute renal failure. *N Engl J Med* 2002;346:305-10.

[129] Bouman CS, Oudemans-Van Straaten HM, Tijssen JG, Zandstra DF, Kese- cioglu J. Effects of early high-volume venovenous hemofiltration on survival and recovery of renal function in intensive care patients with acute renal failure: a prospective, randomised trial. *Crit Care Med* 2002;30:2205-11.

[130] Bent P, Tan HK, Bellomo R, Buckmaster J, Doolan L, Hart G, Silvester W, Gutteridge G, Matalanis G, Raman J, Rosalion A, Buxton BF. Early and intensive continuous hemofiltration for severe renal failure after cardiac surgery. *Ann Thorac Surg* 2001;71:832-7.

[131] Elahi MM, Lim MY, Joseph RN, Dhannapuneni RR, Spyt TJ. Early hemofil- tration improves survival in post-cardiotomy patients with acute renal failure. *Eur J Cardiothorac Surg* 2004;26:1027-31.

[132] Palevsky PM, Zhang JH, O'Connor TZ, Chertow GM, Crowley ST, Choudhry D, Finkel K, Kellum JA, Paganini E, Schein RMH, Smith MW, Swanson KM, Thompson BT, Vijayan A, Watnick S, Star RA, Peduzzi P. Intensity of renal support in critically ill patients with acute kidney injury. *N Engl J Med* 2008;359:1-14.

[133] Tolwani AJ, Campbell RC, Stofan BS, Lai KR, Oster RA, Wille KM. Standard versus high dose CVVHDF for ICU-related acute renal failure. *J Am Soc Nephrol* 2008;19:1233-8.

[134] Kristal B, Shurtz-Swirski R, Tanhilevski O, et al. Epoetin-alpha: preserving kidney function via attenuation of polymorphonuclear leukocyte priming. *Isr Med Assoc J* 2008;10:266-272.

[135] Sutton TA, Kelly KJ, Mang HE, Plotkin Z, Sandoval RM, Dagher PC. Minocycline reduces renal microvascular leakage in a rat model of ischemic renal injury. *Am J Physiol Renal Physiol* 2005;288.

[136] ClinicalTrials.gov. NCT00556491. *Minocycline to prevent acute kidney injury after cardiac surgery.*

[137] Allie DE, Hebert CJ, Walker CM. Multifactorial acute renal failure treated with percutaneous targeted renal therapy (TRT): a case of "dialysis rescue.". *J Invasive Cardiol* 2007;19:E27-E30.

[138] Allie DE, Lirtzman MD, Wyatt CH, et al. Targeted renal therapy and contrast-induced nephropathy during endovascular abdominal aortic aneurysm repair: results of a feasibility pilot trial. *J Endovasc Ther* 2007;14:520-527.

In: Acute Kidney Injury: Causes, Diagnosis and Treatments   ISBN: 978-1-61209-790-9
Editor: Jonathan D. Mendoza, pp. 89-99   © 2011 Nova Science Publishers, Inc.

Chapter VI

Innate and Adaptive Immune Response in Acute Kidney Injury: New Plays in the Play-Offs!

Mariane Tami Amano, Matheus Correa-Costa,
Meire Ioshie Hiyane, Giselle Martins Gonçalves and
Niels Olsen Saraiva Camara[*]

Laboratory of Transplantation Immunobiology. Department of Immunology,
Universidade de São Paulo, São Paulo, Brazil

Abstract

Acute kidney injury (AKI) is the main cause of acute renal failure (ARF) in native
kidneys, being associated with a high mortality and loss of kidney function in the long
term. There are considerable data implicating the important role of the innate and
adaptive immune response in AKI. Toll-like receptor (TLR) are the best-characterized
receptors of innate immunity, able to recognize pathogens associated molecular patterns
(PAMPs), such as LPS, beginning an inflammatory response and also shaping the
adaptive immunity. Endogenous ligands released from damaged or stressed tissues seem
to signal through TLRs. In addition, TLR can activate dendritic cells (DCs). Upon
activation, DCs induce naive T cells to proliferate and polarize to differentiate T helper
subtypes. Recently, another innate immune response receptor, the Nod-like receptors
(NLR), was identified. The role of the NLR in kidney pathologies is less clear but
evidence of its involvement in renal diseases has been reported. Besides, the involvement
of innate immune cells, T cells are also incriminated in the pathogenesis of AKI.
Specifically, CD4+ Th1 cells seem to be the most detrimental. The mechanism of action
of these cells is still on debate; although it seems to involve an antigen-independent
activation. In this review, we will discuss the significance of the innate and adaptive

[*] Address correspondence to: Niels Olsen Saraiva Câmara, M.D., Department of Immunology, Institute of
Biomedical Science IV, Universidade de São Paulo, Prof Lineu Prestes Av, 1730. 05508-900, São Paulo, SP,
Brazil, Phone: (5511) – 3091-7388, Fax: (5511) – 3091-7224, E-mail: niels@icb.usp.br

immune receptors in the development of AKI secondary to different insults such as ischemia and sepsis.

Acute Kidney Injury

Acute kidney injury (AKI) is a clinical condition associated with high levels of morbidity and mortality. Primary renal disease does not usually represent the majority of cases of AKI, but a result of systemic insults such as dehydration, surgery or sepsis leading to renal hypoperfusion. If renal perfusion is not immediately restored, then ischemia reperfusion injury (IRI) can occur in the kidneys leading to acute tubular necrosis (ATN) and functional derangement in the form of AKI [1].

Role of Innate Immunity in Ischemic Acute Kidney Injury

The major cause of morbidity in both allograft and native kidney is the renal IRI [2]. A robust inflammatory response triggered by hypoxia and by the process of reperfusion is determinant for the outcome of the ischemic organ. The presence of inflammatory cytokines and chemokines, an increased expression of adhesion molecules and the recruitment of leukocytes into the post-ischemic kidneys characterize this inflammatory process [3]. Toll-like receptors (TLRs) are transmembrane receptors characterized by an extracellular domain with leucine-rich repeats (LRR) and a TIR (*Toll-interleukin-1 receptor*) intracellular domain, according to its resemblance with interleukin-1 (IL-1) receptors [4]. They are expressed in different cell types such as macrophages, neutrophils, lymphocytes, endothelial and epithelial cells, among other[5]. Recent studies suggest that the TLR-2 and TLR-4 participate in the acute renal injury. Kim *et al.* were the first to show, in a rat model, that after several time of reperfusion after an ischemic injury, the gene and protein expression of TLR-2 and TLR-4 were up-regulated in the kidney tissues [6]. On the other hand, Wu *et al.* showed that HMGB1, Biglycan, HSP70, and HAS-1, -2 and-3 were all upregulated after IRI, implying that they could function as endogenous ligands in this injury model [7].

Studies using genetic modified animals showed that TLR-2, TLR-4 and MyD88 knockout mice were protected from renal IRI, possibly via decreased production of cytokines and chemokines such as IL-1β, IL-6, KC, MCP-1 and diminished neutrophils [7,8,9].

Another subtype of innate immune receptors are the NOD-like receptors (NLRs), a large family comprised of intracellular pattern recognition receptors. Like the TLRs, the NLRs are able to recognize a variety of pathogen-associated molecular patterns and/or danger signals, mediating immune response against pathogen and endogenous damage [10]. The participation of NLR family in the IRI is less clear. Recently, Shigeoka et al. showed expression of Nod-1 and Nod-2 in renal tubular epithelial cells after ischemic injury [11]. They also demonstrated that these receptors were important for the production of pro-inflammatory cytokines such as IL-6, TNF-α and KC.

Independent studies also pointed out the role of inflammasome components in IRI. It has been shown that caspase-1-deficient mice are functionally and histologically protected against

IRI and that this protection is associated with decreased IL-18 in the kidneys [12]. A recent study has also confirmed the pathogenic role of IL-18 in IRI in mice whereas the pretreatment of wild-type mice with IL-18 protein did not protect from damages but the IL-18 deficient mice were protected against IRI [13].

Indeed, the role of IL-1β, and mainly, IL-18, in ATN has been discussed in the last few years. Urinary and serum IL-1β and IL-18 levels have shown to be increased in the urine of patients with ATN and with delayed graft function after transplantation [14].

Role of Innate Immunity in Acute Kidney Injury Triggered by Sepsis

Sepsis results of complex interactions between the infecting microorganism and the inflammatory immune responses from the host. In the United States, the incidence of new cases of sepsis per year is 750,000, with approximately 215,000 deaths [15].

Septic AKI is an important clinical syndrome characterized by abnormal hydroelectrolytic balance and is defined by the simultaneous presence of acute renal failure and sepsis [15]. The limited understanding of the pathophysiology of this disease may possible explain the high incidence of mortality in septic AKI [16].

The understanding of the pathogenesis of septic AKI has been based on the behavior of serum and urinary markers of renal damage. The large amount of experimental data suggests that different cell types and inflammatory mediators are involved in the pathogenesis of organ dysfunction secondary to sepsis [17].

Several studies show the importance of TLRs in the development of sepsis. A work observed that TLR-2 and TLR-4 expression in monocytes from septic patients were significantly increased when compared to expression levels in healthy subjects [18]. Viemann et al. however, observed that the levels of TLR-4 expression in newborns with sepsis were not altered when compared to healthy newborns [19]. Also, another study showed that polymorphonuclear cells and monocytes from patients with sepsis have higher expression of TLR-2 and TLR-4[20]. Brunialti and colleagues [21] observed an increased expression of TLR-4 in monocytes from patients in septic shock while the expression of TLR-2 found unchanged compared to controls. Schaaf et al. [22] also showed that septic patients have increased expression of TLR2 and TLR4 on CD14 monocytes compared with controls and suggest that CD14 and TLR2 are a key factor in monocytes hyporesponsiveness during severe sepsis.

A widely used experimental model of sepsis is the CLP (cecal ligation and puncture), and studies using this model demonstrated that TLR-2 and TLR-4 expression was up regulated in hepatic and splenic macrophages [23] as well as in lungs and in the liver [24]. Andonegui et al. [25] reported an increase of TLR-4 expression, particularly on alveolar endothelial cells, and that lipopolysaccharide (LPS) administration, a TLR4 ligand, played an important role in neutrophils recruitment to the lungs, suggesting that TLR from non-immune cells and immune cells may be involved in tissue injury during sepsis. A recent study showed that the deficiency of neutrophils migration to sites of infection is involved in the pathogenesis of sepsis. Indeed, TLR-4 deficient mice have lower capacity to recruit neutrophils to the inflammatory site after gram-negative sepsis accounting for an increased mortality [26]. These mice also had better survival rates and lower levels of inflammatory cytokines and chemokines in serum [26,27].

The group of Alves-Filho also showed that TLR-2 plays an important role in polymicrobial sepsis and suggested that inhibition of TLR-2 signaling might improve survival in sepsis. TLR-2 knockout mice had lower levels of serum inflammatory cytokines and increased survival rate when compared with wild-type mice [28]. This results are in accordance to studies with patients which showed a decrease in neutrophils migration during sepsis [29,30].

There are few studies showing the involvement of TLRs in septic AKI. A study done by Wolfs *et al.* showed that TLR-2 and TLR-4 are constitutively expressed in epithelial cells of proximal and distal tubules, Bowman's capsule and glomerular epithelium and endothelial cells [31]. It also showed that their expression is increased during the inflammatory process in the presence IFN-γ and TNF-α. These observations suggest that these TLRs may contribute to the activation of immune responses in tubule-interstitial injuries caused by sepsis and other types of renal injury.

Recently, a work also showed that AKI was attenuated in mice deficient in MyD88 but not in TLR-4, and these MyD88-deficient mice do not develop AKI induced by sepsis [32].

The role of NLR family in kidney injuries is even less known, but some studies reported their involvement in kidney diseases and in sepsis. Brenmoehl *et al.* showed that the mortality in septic patients in the ICU was higher in those carrying a NOD-2 frameshift variant [33]. This may represent a consequence of reduced bacterial clearance, leading to enhanced infection and inflammatory cascades, cardiovascular collapse and shock.

Animal and human studies have emphasized the importance of inflammassome pathways in the inflammatory response in sepsis [34]. Caspase-1 knockout mice are protected against *Escherichia coli* endotoxin and from the induction of sepsis [35]. Conversely, a polymorphism that occurs naturally in the human caspase-12, a putative regulator of caspase-1, has been associated with sepsis [36,37].

Caspase-1-deficient mice have higher survival rates and a reduction of renal dysfunction after sepsis and IL-1b and/or IL-18 antagonism was unable to induce renal protection similar to that seen in caspase-1-deficient mice [38]. Also, Caspase-1 deficient mice are protected, whereas IL-1β and Il-1β/IL-18 deficient mice are not protected from endotoxemia [35].

In vivo, mice submitted to LPS treatment showed higher resistance to endotoxic shock in the absence of ASC or NLRP-3. ASC deficient mice tolerated higher doses of LPS compared with NLRP-3 deficient mice, suggesting that ASC is an adapter common to several NLRP molecules [39].

Together, all these data suggest an important role of innate immunity activation on the development of acute kidney injury.

Role of Adaptive Immunity in Ischemic Acute Kidney Injury

Dendritic cells (DCs) are antigen-presenting cells (APC) classically known to activate T cells, which make of DCs a bridge between the innate and adaptive immune response. TLRs are present on DC membranes and the activation of these receptors can lead to DC maturation and modulate T helper cell response [40].

In AKI, endothelial cells facilitates DCs migration to the kidney after ischemia [41] and the number of monocyte derived DCs in the kidney is increased in this situation [42]. After IRI, the expression of MHC class II is increased in monocyte derived DCs as well as the production of IL-12, indicating a mature phenotype [42]. In the same context, DCs are able to induce IFN - γ production by T cells which contributes to the inflammatory process [42]. On the other hand, bone-marrow derived DCs infiltrate kidney, but decrease after IR although their functional activity remains the same [43]. The presence of resident kidney DCs (KDCs) seems to have a major role during the process of IRI. These cells are the main APCs in the kidney and part of them probably migrate to renal lymph nodes after IRI and stimulate T cells [44], which proliferate and produce cytokines that influence the injury and/or repair process. DCs in the kidney produce TNF - □, IL-6, MCP-1 and RANTES and this production increases after IRI insult [45]. Moreover, the predominant secretion of TNF - □ after 24h of reperfusion is done by F4/80^{+ve} KDCs which confirms the importance of these cells during the lesion development [45].

As T cells are known to have a major role in the adaptive immune response 5-7 days after the contact of the pathogen, their participation in AKI is not immediately associated. In the last few years, studies have proved that T cells are not only present [46], but they have an important role during the IRI process. Experiments using double knockout mice for CD4 and CD8 molecules (CD4/CD8$^{-/-}$) [47] or T cells deficient mice (*nu/nu*) [48] did not present IRI as observed in wild-type animals (C57Bl/6). In addition, CD4-deficient and CD4-depleted mice [49] had the same response as the T cells deficient mice, while CD8-deficient mice did not, indicating an important role for CD4$^+$ T cells in the AKI [48]. Another data that corroborates with this idea is that splenic lymphocytes from animals which underwent to IR surgery were transferred to normal mice and after twelve weeks, the latter exhibited increased urinary albumin excretion, meaning that initial AKI predisposes to long-term dysfunction involving T cells [50]. The IRI seems to orientate naïve T cells towards to Th1 response and not Th2. Knockout animals for IL-4 and signal transducers and activators of transcription (STAT)-6, which are associated to a Th2 response, presented a severe renal lesion, while IL-12, IL-12/IFN-□ (double knockout) and STAT4 knockout mice did not present the same damages [51,52,53]. Besides Th1/Th2 modulation, a third T cell population was recently found to be involved in IRI process: the T CD4$^+$CD25$^+$FoxP3$^+$ cells, a well characterized regulatory T cells (Tregs). The presence of these cells was detected into kidneys after ischemic insult and treatment with anti-CD25 (Treg depletion) provoked a worse IRI [54,55,56]. Adoptive transfer of Tregs in wild-type mice improved repair and reduced pro-inflammatory cytokines production [54], while transfer of lymphocytes from Treg deficient mice worsened the renal damage [56]. The protection provided by Tregs in IRI was shown to be IL-10 dependent [56]. However, the whole interaction of Tregs in this model is still a field to be investigated.

T cells activation depends on a first signal that initiates on their TCR. Although it might be expected in AKI, there are only a few studies that demonstrated the involvement of TCR in this model. It was demonstrated that the lack of TCR-□□ conferred injury resistance after ischemia and reperfusion, indicating that this lesion is TCR dependent [57]. Using OVA-TCR-transgenic mice, TCR diversity was shown to be important in IRI, although a limited repertoire is enough to initiate the lesion [58].

All these works suggest that IRI depends on activation of many receptors (TLRs and NLRs) on diverse cell types, especially in APCs as DCs, which consequently interact with T cells making both innate and adaptive immune response work together in the development of the AKI.

Role of Adaptive Immunity in Acute Kidney Injury Triggered by Sepsis

As in IRI, the involvement of adaptive immune cells in septic AKI is still a field to be exploited. In sepsis, the adaptive immune response was thought to occur after the innate response only to prevent new infections, however, many works have shown evidence that adaptive response has an earlier role in sepsis [59].

DCs are one of the cell types that initiate the adaptive immune response. In patients with sepsis, peripheral blood DCs present a profound functional impairment [60], accompanied by a high rate of apoptosis [61]. DC depleted mice present bone marrow-derived DC similar to animals subjected to sepsis by CLP, with an increase in IL-10 production, and a decrease in Th1 priming [62].

Splenic T cells were shown to decrease after CLP [59,63] and it was demonstrated that effector memory T cells are liable to apoptosis [63]. Curiously, septic patients presented Tregs resistant to apoptosis [64]. The ingestion of a large number of apoptotic lymphocytes turns APCs in anti-inflammatory cells [65]. But the role of CD4 T cell remains unclear during early events of sepsis. The mortality of CD4 T cell-deficient mice after CLP is increased in a less severe model (50% 7-day wild-type survival) and no differences were observed in a more severe model (0% 7-day wild-type survival) [66,67]. Many subtypes of T helper cells have been described, as the mentioned above Tregs and the most common Th1 and Th2. Recently, a subtype associated to pro-inflammatory responses was described: Th17, which has the property of produce the IL-17 cytokine. Some authors have already investigated the role of Th17 cells in sepsis and similarly to what was shown with CD4 deficient mice, IL-17R deficient mice had an increase in mortality in a less severe model of CLP, while no differences were observed in the more severe model [68]. Using mouse lines that were known to present a more Th1 or Th2 response, C57Bl6 and Balb/c respectively, the Th2 mouse line had a decrease in survival compared to the Th1 mouse line [69]. These data suggest an important role for T helper cells, mainly in a pro-inflammatory direction, once Th1 and Th-17 are usually associated to inflammatory responses, to combat sepsis. If these cells are also important in the AKI triggered by sepsis, it is still an open question.

In septic AKI, Singbartl and colleagues (2005) [70] demonstrated that the kidney injury was T cells-dependent with CD28 molecule participation. However, this activation was shown to be systemic, once no T cell infiltrated was observed in the kidney. In this work, no APC involvement was investigated, however, they used LPS injection, a TLR4 ligand, to induce sepsis, and we hypothesized that this T cell activation could be done by a DC or macrophage interaction, considering that both have TLR4 and the molecules that bind CD28: CD80 and CD86.

These works demonstrated the involvement of adaptive immune response in sepsis and it is likely that the same occurs in septic AKI, which leaves a wide field to be investigated.

In summary, both innate and adaptive responses are involved in AKI caused by IRI or sepsis. This idea has gained strength in the last few years and it has been shown a complex interaction among different cells and molecules acting in different stages of the injury. Targeting such elements can represent a relevant therapeutic strategy, reducing the disease, and consequently enhancing the patient's quality of life.

References

[1]   Ferenbach DA, Kluth DC, Hughes J Hemeoxygenase-1 and renal ischaemia-reperfusion injury. *Nephron Exp Nephrol* 115: e33-37.

[2]   Thadhani R, Pascual M, Bonventre JV (1996) Acute renal failure. *N Engl J Med* 334: 1448-1460.

[3]   Bonventre JV, Zuk A (2004) Ischemic acute renal failure: an inflammatory disease? *Kidney Int* 66: 480-485.

[4]   Medzhitov R (2001) Toll-like receptors and innate immunity. *Nat Rev Immunol* 1: 135-145.

[5]   Akira S, Uematsu S, Takeuchi O (2006) Pathogen recognition and innate immunity. *Cell* 124: 783-801.

[6]   Kim BS, Lim SW, Li C, Kim JS, Sun BK, et al. (2005) Ischemia-reperfusion injury activates innate immunity in rat kidneys. *Transplantation* 79: 1370-1377.

[7]   Wu H, Chen G, Wyburn KR, Yin J, Bertolino P, et al. (2007) TLR4 activation mediates kidney ischemia/reperfusion injury. *J Clin Invest* 117: 2847-2859.

[8]   Pulskens WP, Teske GJ, Butter LM, Roelofs JJ, van der Poll T, et al. (2008) Toll-like receptor-4 coordinates the innate immune response of the kidney to renal ischemia/reperfusion injury. *PLoS One* 3: e3596.

[9]   Rusai K, Sollinger D, Baumann M, Wagner B, Strobl M, et al. Toll-like receptors 2 and 4 in renal ischemia/reperfusion injury. *Pediatr Nephrol* 25: 853-860.

[10]   Jin C, Flavell RA Molecular mechanism of NLRP3 inflammasome activation. *J Clin Immunol* 30: 628-631.

[11]   Shigeoka AA, Kambo A, Mathison JC, King AJ, Hall WF, et al. Nod1 and nod2 are expressed in human and murine renal tubular epithelial cells and participate in renal ischemia reperfusion injury. *J Immunol* 184: 2297-2304.

[12]   Melnikov VY, Ecder T, Fantuzzi G, Siegmund B, Lucia MS, et al. (2001) Impaired IL-18 processing protects caspase-1-deficient mice from ischemic acute renal failure. *J Clin Invest* 107: 1145-1152.

[13]   Wu H, Craft ML, Wang P, Wyburn KR, Chen G, et al. (2008) IL-18 contributes to renal damage after ischemia-reperfusion. *J Am Soc Nephrol* 19: 2331-2341.

[14]   Parikh CR, Jani A, Melnikov VY, Faubel S, Edelstein CL (2004) Urinary interleukin-18 is a marker of human acute tubular necrosis. *Am J Kidney Dis* 43: 405-414.

[15]   Angus DC, Linde-Zwirble WT, Lidicker J, Clermont G, Carcillo J, et al. (2001) Epidemiology of severe sepsis in the United States: analysis of incidence, outcome, and associated costs of care. *Crit Care Med* 29: 1303-1310.

[16]   Bellomo R, Wan L, Langenberg C, May C (2008) Septic acute kidney injury: new concepts. *Nephron Exp Nephrol* 109: e95-100.

[17] Russell JA (2006) Management of sepsis. *N Engl J Med* 355: 1699-1713.

[18] Armstrong L, Medford AR, Hunter KJ, Uppington KM, Millar AB (2004) Differential expression of Toll-like receptor (TLR)-2 and TLR-4 on monocytes in human sepsis. *Clin Exp Immunol* 136: 312-319.

[19] Viemann D, Dubbel G, Schleifenbaum S, Harms E, Sorg C, et al. (2005) Expression of toll-like receptors in neonatal sepsis. *Pediatr Res* 58: 654-659.

[20] Harter L, Mica L, Stocker R, Trentz O, Keel M (2004) Increased expression of toll-like receptor-2 and -4 on leukocytes from patients with sepsis. *Shock* 22: 403-409.

[21] Brunialti MK, Martins PS, Barbosa de Carvalho H, Machado FR, Barbosa LM, et al. (2006) TLR2, TLR4, CD14, CD11B, and CD11C expressions on monocytes surface and cytokine production in patients with sepsis, severe sepsis, and septic shock. *Shock* 25: 351-357.

[22] Schaaf B, Luitjens K, Goldmann T, van Bremen T, Sayk F, et al. (2009) Mortality in human sepsis is associated with downregulation of Toll-like receptor 2 and CD14 expression on blood monocytes. *Diagn Pathol* 4: 12.

[23] Tsujimoto H, Ono S, Majima T, Kawarabayashi N, Takayama E, et al. (2005) Neutrophil elastase, MIP-2, and TLR-4 expression during human and experimental sepsis. *Shock* 23: 39-44.

[24] Williams DL, Ha T, Li C, Kalbfleisch JH, Schweitzer J, et al. (2003) Modulation of tissue Toll-like receptor 2 and 4 during the early phases of polymicrobial sepsis correlates with mortality. *Crit Care Med* 31: 1808-1818.

[25] Andonegui G, Bonder CS, Green F, Mullaly SC, Zbytnuik L, et al. (2003) Endothelium-derived Toll-like receptor-4 is the key molecule in LPS-induced neutrophil sequestration into lungs. *J Clin Invest* 111: 1011-1020.

[26] Alves-Filho JC, Tavares-Murta BM, Barja-Fidalgo C, Benjamim CF, Basile-Filho A, et al. (2006) Neutrophil function in severe sepsis. *Endocr Metab Immune Disord Drug Targets* 6: 151-158.

[27] Alves-Filho JC, de Freitas A, Russo M, Cunha FQ (2006) Toll-like receptor 4 signaling leads to neutrophil migration impairment in polymicrobial sepsis. *Crit Care Med* 34: 461-470.

[28] Alves-Filho JC, Freitas A, Souto FO, Spiller F, Paula-Neto H, et al. (2009) Regulation of chemokine receptor by Toll-like receptor 2 is critical to neutrophil migration and resistance to polymicrobial sepsis. *Proc Natl Acad Sci U S A* 106: 4018-4023.

[29] Chishti AD, Shenton BK, Kirby JA, Baudouin SV (2004) Neutrophil chemotaxis and receptor expression in clinical septic shock. *Intensive Care Med* 30: 605-611.

[30] Tavares-Murta BM, Zaparoli M, Ferreira RB, Silva-Vergara ML, Oliveira CH, et al. (2002) Failure of neutrophil chemotactic function in septic patients. *Crit Care Med* 30: 1056-1061.

[31] Wolfs TG, Buurman WA, van Schadewijk A, de Vries B, Daemen MA, et al. (2002) In vivo expression of Toll-like receptor 2 and 4 by renal epithelial cells: IFN-gamma and TNF-alpha mediated up-regulation during inflammation. *J Immunol* 168: 1286-1293.

[32] Dear JW, Yasuda H, Hu X, Hieny S, Yuen PS, et al. (2006) Sepsis-induced organ failure is mediated by different pathways in the kidney and liver: acute renal failure is dependent on MyD88 but not renal cell apoptosis. *Kidney Int* 69: 832-836.

[33] Brenmoehl J, Herfarth H, Gluck T, Audebert F, Barlage S, et al. (2007) Genetic variants in the NOD2/CARD15 gene are associated with early mortality in sepsis patients. Intensive *Care Med* 33: 1541-1548.

[34] Scott AM, Saleh M (2007) The inflammatory caspases: guardians against infections and sepsis. *Cell Death Differ* 14: 23-31.

[35] Sarkar A, Hall MW, Exline M, Hart J, Knatz N, et al. (2006) Caspase-1 regulates Escherichia coli sepsis and splenic B cell apoptosis independently of interleukin-1beta and interleukin-18. *Am J Respir Crit Care Med* 174: 1003-1010.

[36] Saleh M, Mathison JC, Wolinski MK, Bensinger SJ, Fitzgerald P, et al. (2006) Enhanced bacterial clearance and sepsis resistance in caspase-12-deficient mice. *Nature* 440: 1064-1068.

[37] Saleh M, Vaillancourt JP, Graham RK, Huyck M, Srinivasula SM, et al. (2004) Differential modulation of endotoxin responsiveness by human caspase-12 polymorphisms. *Nature* 429: 75-79.

[38] Babelova A, Moreth K, Tsalastra-Greul W, Zeng-Brouwers J, Eickelberg O, et al. (2009) Biglycan, a danger signal that activates the NLRP3 inflammasome via toll-like and P2X receptors. *J Biol Chem* 284: 24035-24048.

[39] Sutterwala FS, Ogura Y, Szczepanik M, Lara-Tejero M, Lichtenberger GS, et al. (2006) Critical role for NALP3/CIAS1/Cryopyrin in innate and adaptive immunity through its regulation of caspase-1. *Immunity* 24: 317-327.

[40] Jakob T, Walker PS, Krieg AM, Udey MC, Vogel JC (1998) Activation of cutaneous dendritic cells by CpG-containing oligodeoxynucleotides: a role for dendritic cells in the augmentation of Th1 responses by immunostimulatory DNA. *J Immunol* 161: 3042-3049.

[41] Schlichting CL, Schareck WD, Weis M (2006) Renal ischemia-reperfusion injury: new implications of dendritic cell-endothelial cell interactions. *Transplant Proc* 38: 670-673.

[42] Wu CJ, Sheu JR, Chen HH, Liao HF, Yang YC, et al. (2006) Modulation of monocyte-derived dendritic cell differentiation is associated with ischemic acute renal failure. *J Surg Res* 132: 104-111.

[43] Wu CJ, Sheu JR, Chen HH, Liao HF, Yang YC, et al. (2006) Renal ischemia/reperfusion injury inhibits differentiation of dendritic cells derived from bone marrow monocytes in rats. *Life Sci* 78: 1121-1128.

[44] Dong X, Swaminathan S, Bachman LA, Croatt AJ, Nath KA, et al. (2005) Antigen presentation by dendritic cells in renal lymph nodes is linked to systemic and local injury to the kidney. *Kidney Int* 68: 1096-1108.

[45] Dong X, Swaminathan S, Bachman LA, Croatt AJ, Nath KA, et al. (2007) Resident dendritic cells are the predominant TNF-secreting cell in early renal ischemia-reperfusion injury. *Kidney Int* 71: 619-628.

[46] Ysebaert DK, De Greef KE, Vercauteren SR, Ghielli M, Verpooten GA, et al. (2000) Identification and kinetics of leukocytes after severe ischaemia/reperfusion renal injury. *Nephrol Dial Transplant* 15: 1562-1574.

[47] . Rabb H, Daniels F, O'Donnell M, Haq M, Saba SR, et al. (2000) Pathophysiological role of T lymphocytes in renal ischemia-reperfusion injury in mice. *Am J Physiol Renal Physiol* 279: F525-531.

[48] Burne MJ, Daniels F, El Ghandour A, Mauiyyedi S, Colvin RB, et al. (2001) Identification of the CD4(+) T cell as a major pathogenic factor in ischemic acute renal failure. *J Clin Invest* 108: 1283-1290.

[49] Pinheiro HS, Camara NO, Noronha IL, Maugeri IL, Franco MF, et al. (2007) Contribution of CD4+ T cells to the early mechanisms of ischemia- reperfusion injury in a mouse model of acute renal failure. *Braz J Med Biol Res* 40: 557-568.

[50] Burne-Taney MJ, Liu M, Ascon D, Molls RR, Racusen L, et al. (2006) Transfer of lymphocytes from mice with renal ischemia can induce albuminuria in naive mice: a possible mechanism linking early injury and progressive renal disease? *Am J Physiol Renal Physiol* 291: F981-986.

[51] Yokota N, Burne-Taney M, Racusen L, Rabb H (2003) Contrasting roles for STAT4 and STAT6 signal transduction pathways in murine renal ischemia-reperfusion injury. *Am J Physiol Renal Physiol* 285: F319-325.

[52] de Paiva VN, Monteiro RM, Marques Vde P, Cenedeze MA, Teixeira Vde P, et al. (2009) Critical involvement of Th1-related cytokines in renal injuries induced by ischemia and reperfusion. *Int Immunopharmacol* 9: 668-672.

[53] Marques VP, Goncalves GM, Feitoza CQ, Cenedeze MA, Fernandes Bertocchi AP, et al. (2006) Influence of TH1/TH2 switched immune response on renal ischemia-reperfusion injury. *Nephron Exp Nephrol* 104: e48-56.

[54] Gandolfo MT, Jang HR, Bagnasco SM, Ko GJ, Agreda P, et al. (2009) Foxp3+ regulatory T cells participate in repair of ischemic acute kidney injury. *Kidney Int* 76: 717-729.

[55] Monteiro RM, Camara NO, Rodrigues MM, Tzelepis F, Damiao MJ, et al. (2009) A role for regulatory T cells in renal acute kidney injury. *Transpl Immunol* 21: 50-55.

[56] Kinsey GR, Sharma R, Huang L, Li L, Vergis AL, et al. (2009) Regulatory T cells suppress innate immunity in kidney ischemia-reperfusion injury. *J Am Soc Nephrol* 20: 1744-1753.

[57] Hochegger K, Schatz T, Eller P, Tagwerker A, Heininger D, et al. (2007) Role of alpha/beta and gamma/delta T cells in renal ischemia-reperfusion injury. *Am J Physiol Renal Physiol* 293: F741-747.

[58] Satpute SR, Park JM, Jang HR, Agreda P, Liu M, et al. (2009) The role for T cell repertoire/antigen-specific interactions in experimental kidney ischemia reperfusion injury. *J Immunol* 183: 984-992.

[59] Kasten KR, Tschop J, Adediran SG, Hildeman DA, Caldwell CC T cells are potent early mediators of the host response to sepsis. *Shock* 34: 327-336.

[60] Poehlmann H, Schefold JC, Zuckermann-Becker H, Volk HD, Meisel C (2009) Phenotype changes and impaired function of dendritic cell subsets in patients with sepsis: a prospective observational analysis. *Crit Care* 13: R119.

[61] Riccardi F, Della Porta MG, Rovati B, Casazza A, Radolovich D, et al. Flow cytometric analysis of peripheral blood dendritic cells in patients with severe sepsis. *Cytometry B Clin Cytom* 80: 14-21.

[62] Pastille E, Didovic S, Brauckmann D, Rani M, Agrawal H, et al. Modulation of dendritic cell differentiation in the bone marrow mediates sustained immun-osuppression after polymicrobial sepsis. *J Immunol* 186: 977-986.

[63] McDunn JE, Turnbull IR, Polpitiya AD, Tong A, MacMillan SK, et al. (2006) Splenic CD4+ T cells have a distinct transcriptional response six hours after the onset of sepsis. *J Am Coll Surg* 203: 365-375.

[64] Venet F, Chung CS, Kherouf H, Geeraert A, Malcus C, et al. (2009) Increased circulating regulatory T cells (CD4(+)CD25 (+)CD127 (-)) contribute to lymphocyte anergy in septic shock patients. *Intensive Care Med* 35: 678-686.

[65] Voll RE, Herrmann M, Roth EA, Stach C, Kalden JR, et al. (1997) Immunosuppressive effects of apoptotic cells. *Nature* 390: 350-351.

[66] Martignoni A, Tschop J, Goetzman HS, Choi LG, Reid MD, et al. (2008) CD4-expressing cells are early mediators of the innate immune system during sepsis. *Shock* 29: 591-597.

[67] Enoh VT, Lin SH, Etogo A, Lin CY, Sherwood ER (2008) CD4+ T-cell depletion is not associated with alterations in survival, bacterial clearance, and inflammation after cecal ligation and puncture. *Shock* 29: 56-64.

[68] Freitas A, Alves-Filho JC, Victoni T, Secher T, Lemos HP, et al. (2009) IL-17 receptor signaling is required to control polymicrobial sepsis. *J Immunol* 182: 7846-7854.

[69] Watanabe H, Numata K, Ito T, Takagi K, Matsukawa A (2004) Innate immune response in Th1- and Th2-dominant mouse strains. Shock 22: 460-466.

[70] Singbartl K, Bockhorn SG, Zarbock A, Schmolke M, Van Aken H (2005) T cells modulate neutrophil-dependent acute renal failure during endotoxemia: critical role for CD28. *J Am Soc Nephrol 16: 720-728.*

In: Acute Kidney Injury: Causes, Diagnosis and Treatments   ISBN: 978-1-61209-790-9
Editor: Jonathan D. Mendoza, pp. 101-109   © 2011 Nova Science Publishers, Inc.

Chapter VII

Pandemic H1N1 Influenza A Infection and Acute Kidney Injury

*David Collister, Irfan Moledina, Katie Pundyk, Kerrett Wallace and Manish M Sood**

University of Manitoba, Winnipeg, Manitoba, Canada

Abstract

The recent global outbreak of pandemic H1N1 (pH1N1) influenza A infection strained global intensive care unit resources as critically ill patients often required respiratory support. Early data suggests a large proportion of patients suffered acute kidney injury and required renal replacement therapy. This review will outline the impact of the pH1N1 outbreak, discuss the epidemiology and mechanisms of acute kidney injury due to pH1N1, and suggest general treatment recommendations.

Introduction

As the global influenza A (pH1N1) pandemic concludes, we can begin to thoroughly investigate the magnitude of its effect on the population and healthcare resources. The major concern with the pH1N1 pandemic was reports concerning significantly increased morbidity and mortality in young otherwise healthy adults in Mexico [1]. As the infection spread globally, it became apparent mortality rates were not as high as initially perceived. Nevertheless a large number of young, healthy adults required hospital admission and respiratory support due to the infection. Acute kidney injury (AKI) with or with out the need for subsequent dialysis therapy is strongly associated with mortality and early reports suggest it is common in patients with severe pH1N1 [2]. In this review, we will discuss the impact of

* University of Manitoba, 409 Tache Avenue, Winnipeg, Manitoba, R2H 2A6, Tel: 204-237-2121, FAX: 204-233-27

pH1N1 infection on AKI, explore possible mechanisms of injury and suggest general management strategies and treatment possibilities for infected patients.

An Introduction to pH1N1

Pandemic influenza A (H1N1) can cause an influenza-like-illness (ILI) defined by Centers for Disease Control and Prevention as a fever (temperature $\geq 37.8°C$ or $100°F$) and a cough and/or sore throat in the absence of a known cause other than influenza [3]. In order to test a case of ILI for the pandemic influenza A (H1N1) virus a real-time reverse transcriptase (RT) - PCR for influenza A, B, H1, and H3 is done[4]. Pandemic influenza A (H1N1) has been identified as the cause of the 'Spanish' influenza pandemic from 1918 – 1919. The mortality rate was up to 50 million worldwide, with a relatively high mortality rate in young adults compared to other pandemics [5]. The influenza virus can evolve in two different ways, defined as antigenic drift and antigenic shift. 'Drift' applies to the virus that acquires point mutations over time while 'shift' involves a larger change in the viral genes [6]. These episodes are thought to be descendants of the 1918 virus and can be considered 'shift' pandemics [7]. Influenza can be difficult to control because a person could potentially transmit the virus before becoming ill and up to 7 days after their illness. H1N1 is thought to be transferred from person to person through large-particle droplet transmission. The droplets are thought to travel no more than 6 feet between people. H1N1 may also be transmitted from contaminated surfaces or through small-droplet nuclei ('airborne') [8]. The pandemic influenza A (H1N1) has spread more quickly than other pandemics. In previous pandemics it has taken more than six months to spread as widely as it has in less than 6 weeks [9]. This is likely a result of airline travel [10]. The pandemic influenza A (H1N1) virus has affected people from age 3 months to 81 years. 60% of these are 18 years old or younger, which is similar to the seasonal influenza [11]. The average age of cases is 12 – 17 years old, although it may be that older individuals have an increased rate of hospitalization and mortality. In some countries there is the seasonal influenza as well as the pandemic influenza A (H1N1) so it is difficult to tell the exact morbidity and mortality of the different age ranges [12].

The mortality associated with pandemic influenza A (H1N1) in the elderly has not occurred to the extent expected when compared to seasonal influenza. It has been suggested that this could be due to an immunity acquired from a virus that was present before 1957[13]. It has been shown that the survivors of the 1918 influenza pandemic have 'viral-neutralizing antibodies' still present in their system [14]. Despite this advantage in the elderly it has been found that during influenza pandemics in the USA around 50% of the deaths occurred in people less than 65 years old; then in the epidemics over the next decade the rate of deaths fell in the age group less than 65 and increased in the group above 65[15].

High risk groups are people more likely to suffer complications when acquiring pandemic influenza A (H1N1). These groups are considered to be the same for pandemic influenza A (H1N1) as for the seasonal influenza virus. The groups are children <5 years old, adults ≥65 years old, people with chronic pulmonary, cardiovascular, renal, hepatic, hematological, neurologic, neuromuscular, or metabolic disorders, immunosuppression, pregnant women, people <19 years old on long-term aspirin therapy, and residents of nursing homes or chronic-care facilities[8].

Influenza A H1N1 and Acute Kidney Injury

There is only a paucity of literature reporting the impact of pH1N1 and AKI with the focus on renal injury in the critically ill [2, 16, 17]. Critically ill patients with H1N1 influenza A virus who develop AKI are at increased risk of mortality, length of hospital/ICU stay and the development of CKD(2). ARDS and hypoxemic respiratory failure is the focus of care in these critically ill patients but the development of AKI and its incidence, natural history, risk factors and treatment is of increasing relevance. Unfortunately, only a few studies have examined these factors. A cohort study of 50 H1N1 patients (72% women, 48% aboriginal, BMI 34.8 +/- 12.0kg/m^2) with ICU admissions for ventilatory support in Manitoba, Canada is the initial study of its kind to evaluate these issues. AKI was seen in 66.7% of patients with 22% requiring renal replacement therapy (RRT). Of these RRT patients, 22% died, 11% required continuous RRT and the remaining recovered renal function. Patients with advanced age, elevated BMI and a history of asthma were at increased risk of developing AKI.

Another study examined 22 patients with H1N1 influenza pneumonia admitted to the ICU (age 52.91 +/- 18.89 years; 50% male). 63.6% developed AKI with 18.2% needing RRT with a mean duration of 15 +/- 12 days [18]. 42.9 % recovered renal function. AKI was associated with pregnancy, immunosuppression, high APACHE, SOFA and MURRAY scores, less time on mechanical ventilation assistance, hemodynamic instability and thrombocytopenia. Hemodialysis requirements were associated with elevated SOFA scores, elevated creatine phosphokinase and alanine transferase levels.

These early studies have led to some noteworthy observations. Firstly, the reported rates of AKI in critically ill pH1N1 are surprisingly high considering this is a young ICU population with little co-morbidity. It has been speculated that higher immune competency in young adults leads to a more severe systemic inflammatory response with resultant end organ damage. Secondly, patients with AKI had high requirements for dialysis therapy and required longer, more resource intensive ICU admissions. If the pandemic were as severe as initially anticipated, this would have profound impacts on worldwide ICU resources. Thirdly, although the majority of patients with AKI did not require permanent dialysis therapy, it remains unclear if this predisposes them to premature renal injury in the future.

Mechanisms of Kidney Injury with pH1N1

The mechanism of renal injury by the H1N1 influenza A virus although unclear, appears to be multifactorial. AKI in the setting of respiratory virus infections is not uncommon; several case studies and series exist that describe AKI secondary to influenza A, B, H5N1, parainfluenza and SARS-associated coronavirus infections and virus-induced rhabdomyolysis [19-24]. Influenza A is also thought to cause AKI by mechanisms other than rhabdomyolysis including renal hypoperfusion from viral sepsis, the development of DIC and microvascular insults as well as MODS [25].

Case studies have recently reported AKI in the setting of Influenza A H1N1 secondary to rhabdomyolysis in pediatric and adult patients [23, 26]. However, the pathogenesis of virus-induced rhabdomyolysis is poorly understood. It is thought to involve viral invasion of muscle fibres leading to lymphocytic infiltration, phagocytosis, cellular injury, necrosis of myofibrils and muscle fibre degeneration [21]. Studies support this theory as tissue cultures of muscle fibres in patients with rhabomyolysis and Influenza A infection has grown the virus although no virus has been visualized on electron microscopy (EM) [27]. Myoglobin from injured muscle fibres becomes concentrated along renal tubules, a process that is enhanced by volume depletion and renal vasoconstriction, and precipitates through interactions with the Tamm-Horsfall protein leading to intrarenal vasoconstriction, direct and ischemic tubule injury and tubular obstruction. An elevated serum CK is the most sensitive marker of muscle injury but has not been shown to be predictive of patients at increased risk of AKI [22] There is no defined threshold value above which the risk of AKI is markedly increased and the risk of AKI in rhabdomyolysis is usually low when CK levels at admission are less than 15000-20000 U/L. However, AKI may be associated with CK values as low as 5000 U/L, this usually occurs with coexisting conditions such as sepsis, dehydration and acidosis.

The prognosis for myoglobinuria-associated ARF is generally good, with the majority of patients regaining full kidney function within weeks to months [22]. Direct viral infiltration of the kidney by the H1N1 influenza virus may also contribute to AKI with infection of respiratory epithelial cells extending to immune cells and renal epithelial cells. This is similar to a proposed mechanism of renal injury in SARS after in-situ hybridization and electro microscopy revealed affinity of viral particles to the distal tubules of the kidney [28].However, no studies examining the renal tropism of the influenza H1N1 virus have been completed in humans. Mouse models do not support this theory as the virus has not been isolated in the kidney by means of tissue culture or EM.

The role of SIRS/MODS in the pathogenesis of AKI with H1N1 influenza A infection is also unclear. The "slippery slope" of critical illness and its associated inflammatory cytokines, tissue hypoxia, reactive oxygen species, ischemic reperfusion injury and DIC, all which may impact renal function in critically ill patients [25]. Mechanical ventilation and its effects on renal function through hemodynamic disturbances (reduction in cardiac output, redistribution of renal blood flow (RBF), stimulation of hormonal and sympathetic pathways), blood gas effects (hypoxemic and hypercapnic alterations in RBF) and biotraumatic release of inflammatory cytokines may also play a role [29].

Goodpasture's Syndrome has also been associated with Influenza A2 virus infection with the theory that pulmonary infection may induce a patient to form antibodies reactive to glomerular basement membranes, either by causing an antigenic alteration of the basement membrane causing it to become immunogenic or by acting as an adjuvant and enhancing the immunogenicity [30]. The mechanism of renal injury by the H1N1 influenza A virus is still unknown but is thought to be multifactorial in the critical care setting. Studies that explore virus-induced rhabdomyolysis and the critical care setting as etiologic factors AKI with corresponding renal and muscle histology, viral cultures and EM are needed to further delineate its pathophysiology.

The Immune System in Uremia

Infection is a frequent complication and cause of death in renal failure. Although it is widely accepted that uremia has an adverse effect on host resistance to infectious disease this immune dysfunction is not fully understood. It is postulated that uremic patients have a high infectious morbidity, likely due to a complex interaction between the innate and adaptive systems in which immune activation and immune suppression coexist, with resultant deficient responses of T lymphocytes and significantly depressed specific antibody responses [31]. Interestingly, the main cause of death in patients with chronic kidney disease remains cardiovascular and infectious diseases both being pathological processes associated with immune dysfunction (chronic inflammation with accelerated tissue degeneration and poorly orchestrated immune response).

The susceptibility to both bacterial and viral infections in uremic patients appears multifactorial. Patients on intermittent hemodialysis and continuous ambulatory peritoneal dialysis have a diminished polymorphonuclear leukocyte function with impairment seen in chemotaxis, phagocytosis, intracellular killing by proteolytic enzymes and production of toxic oxygen radicals. Also contributing to this dysfunction is iron overload, elevated levels of intracellular calcium and hemodialysis treatment itself. Uremic patients also have elevated levels of glucose-modified serum proteins and free immunoglobulin light chains (IgLCs). The former increases chemotactic movement of neutrophils and the later increases the percentage of viable neutrophils by inhibiting spontaneous apoptotic cell death. As a result both modulate and contribute to the disturbed immune function.

Experiments have shown a reduce capacity of monocytes to synthesize proinflammatory cytokines (TNF-alpha, IL-1 beta, IL-6 and IL-8) in response to lipopolysaccharide stimulation in patients with chronic kidney disease (31). This is thought to be due to reduced monocyte expression of Toll-like receptors (TLR) making this cohort of patients more susceptible to bacterial infections.

The summative result of all of these perturbations in immunity in the uremic state is the increased susceptibility to acquiring new infections and the inability to mount an adequate host response to an established infection or other immune stimulus, such as vaccination [32].

Treatment of pH1N1 in End Stage Renal Disease

Most strains of swine H1N1 influenza A virus circulating appear to be sensitive *in vitro* to the neuraminidase inhibitors (oseltamivir and zanamivir) but resistant to amantadine and rimantadine [32, 33]. Recently isolated cases of resistance to oseltamivir have been reported [34, 35].

Antiviral therapy is recommended for all hospitalized patients with confirmed or suspected H1N1 influenza A virus infection and patients at increased risk for complications [8]. Patients with mild illness may or may not need to be treated however this is based on the clinician's judgment. Therapy should be started immediately as greater benefit has been demonstrated with early initiation of treatment, preferably within 48 hours of onset of illness as seen with seasonal influenza.

It is also recommended that close contacts who are at a high risk for complications of influenza (patients with chronic medical conditions, > 65yrs of age, pregnant women) receive post-exposure antiviral prophylaxis [9]. In addition health care workers, public health workers, first responders who did not use appropriate personal protective equipment should be treated. Pre-exposure antiviral prophylaxis is limited to individuals who have ongoing occupational risk for exposure. Prophylaxis should be continued for ten days after the last know exposure to a patient with confirmed H1N1 influenza A. No prophylaxis is needed if contact occurred outside of the infectious period (one day before until seven days after onset of illness).

Treatment for novel H1N1 influenza A virus infection in patients with normal renal function is oseltamivir 75mg orally twice a day for five days. Oseltamivir is renally eliminated and thereby should be reduced to 75mg orally 3 times a week in ESRD and can be dosed after hemodialysis [35]. Alternatively, doses of 30 mg daily have been shown to achieve adequate clinical exposure of the active form of the drug and may be used as an alternative [36]. Zanamivir is also available however little data exists on renal dosing adjustments.

Oseltamivir and zanamivir are pregnancy category C drugs however pregnant women have a greater propensity for severe disease hence therapy should not be withheld (potential benefit outweighs the theoretical risk to the fetus) [8, 35]. Oseltamivir is preferentially used because of its systemic absorption. Patients admitted to hospital with superimposed bacterial infections should be treated with empiric antibiotic agents. Vaccination is recommended for pregnant women, healthcare and emergency medical services personnel, household contacts and caregivers for children younger than 6 months of age, all people from 6 months old through 24 years of age, and persons age 25 through 64 years who have health conditions associated with higher risk of medical complications from influenza.

Influenza A/ H1N1 is transmitted by aersolization of respiratory droplet particles posing a unique problem in the close quarters encountered in many hemodialysis units. These guidelines apply to the health care workers in all health care settings inclusive of hospital care, acute care, long term care, ambulatory care, physician offices, community setting and home care. As such, routine practices, such as droplet and contact precautions are appropriate measures for care of individuals with Influenza- Like illness (fever>38 C and cough and one or more of sore throat, rhinorrhea, nasal congestion, arthralgia, myalgia or prostration), suspected or confirmed H1N1 influenza A virus.

Routine practices/ contact precautions are done to prevent transmission of microorganisms between patients and between the health care worker and patients. This involves stringent hand hygiene (use of alcohol based hand sanitizer/ soap and water before and after contact with patients , body fluids or equipment), cough etiquette (cough into sleeve), use of personal protective equipment (disposable glove, gown, N95 respirator mask, eye and facial protection with goggles/ facial shield) and lastly, patient management issues.

Isolation precautions are enforced for seven days after onset of symptoms or until asymptomatic (no fever, myalgia, arthralgia, sore throat, productive cough) whichever is longer for suspected or confirmed cases. Isolation rooms should clearly be identified as contact/droplet precautions. For aerosol-generating activities such as endotracheal intubation, nebulizations, bronchoscopy an airborne isolation room with negative pressure air handling with 6 to 12 air changes per hour is ideal. Health personnel involved in care should wear a fit-tested N95 respirator.

A high degree of suspicion of infection is required in the end stage renal disease population as the clinical presentation may be atypical [37]. Wiebe et al. reported an atypical case of pH1N1 that was misdiagnosed as volume overload and congestive heart failure. This resulted in the lack of appropriate precautions being taken and numerous other hemodialysis patients being exposed.

Conclusion

H1N1 influenza A has allowed unique insights into the impact of a viral pandemic on renal disease and injury. Although truncated in its severity, early reports suggest a high rate of kidney injury and the need for dialysis therapies among the critically ill. The mechanism of renal injury seems to involve the merger of multiple pathways of injury. In uremic patients, immune dysfunction would increase susceptibility to infection thereby necessitating appropriate infection control practices and timely treatment with anti-virals.

References

[1]   Centre for Disease Control: Outbreak of swine-origin influenza A (H1N1) virus infection - Mexico, March-April 2009. *MMWR Morb. Mortal. Wkly. Rep.* 2009; 58: 467-470.

[2]   Manish MS, Claudio R, Ryan Z, Paul K, *et al.* Acute Kidney Injury in Critically Ill Patients Infected With 2009 Pandemic Influenza A(H1N1): Report From a Canadian Province. *American Journal of Kidney Diseases: The Official Journal of the National Kidney Foundation* 55: 848-855.

[3]   Centre for Disease Control: Interim guidance on specimen collection, processing, and testing for patients with suspected swine-origin influenza A (H1N1) virus infection. In, June 2009.

[4]   Centre for Disease Control: Interim guidance on case definitions to be used for investigations of novel influenza A (H1N1) cases in 2009.

[5]   Novel Swine-Origin Influenza AVIT. Emergence of a Novel Swine-Origin Influenza A (H1N1) Virus in Humans. *N. Engl. J. Med.* 2009; 360: 2605-2615.

[6]   CW O. The emergence of novel swine influenza viruses in North America. *Virus Res.* 2002; 85: 199-210.

[7]   Morens DM TJ, Fauci AS. The persistent legacy of the 1918 influenza virus. *NEJM* 2009; 361: 225-229.

[8]   Centre for Disease Control: Interim guidance on antiviral recommendations for patients with novel influenza A (H1N1) virus infection and their close contacts. In (vol 2009), 2009

[9]   Centre for Disease Control: Interim guidance for clinicians on identifying and caring for patient swith swine-origin influenza A (H1N1) infection. In (vol 2009).

[10]   Khan K AJ, Hu W, Raposo P, Sears J, Calderon F, et al. Spread of a novel influenza A (H1N1) virus via global airline transportation. . *NEJM* 2009; 361: 212-214.

[11]   WHO: Pandemic (H1N1) 2009 - update 59. In (vol 2009), 2009.

[12]   WHO: Preliminary information important for understanding the evolving situation In (vol 2009), 2009.

[13]   Centre for Disease Control: H1N1 spreads about as readily as seasonal flu, May 20, 2009 In (vol 2009), 2009.

[14]   Yu X TT, McGraw PA, House FS, Keefer CJ, Hicar MD, et al. Neutralizing antibodies derived from the B cells of 1918 influenza pandemic survivors. *Nature* 2008; 455: 532-536.

[15] Simonsen L CM, Schonberger LB, Arden NH, Cox NJ, Fukuda K. . Pandemic versus epidemic influenza mortality: A pattern of changing age distribution. . *J. Infect. Dis.* 1998; 178: 53-60.

[16] Jain S, Kamimoto L, Bramley AM, Schmitz AM, *et al.* Hospitalized Patients with 2009 H1N1 Influenza in the United States, April-June 2009. *N. Engl. J. Med.* 2009: NEJMoa0906695.

[17] Kumar A, Zarychanski R, Pinto R, Cook DJ, *et al.* Critically Ill Patients With 2009 Influenza A(H1N1) Infection in Canada. *JAMA* 2009; 302: 1872-1879.

[18] Trimarchi H GG, Campolo-Girard V, Giannasi S, Pomeranz V, San-Roman E, Lombi F, Barcan L, Forrester M, Algranati S, Iriarte R, Rosa-Diez G. H1N1 infection and the kidney in critically ill patients. *J. Nephrol.* 2010.

[19] Chu KH, Tsang WK, Tang CS, Lam MF, *et al.* Acute renal impairment in coronavirus-associated severe acute respiratory syndrome. *Kidney Int.* 2005; 67: 698-705.

[20] Fowler RA, Lapinsky SE, Hallett D, Detsky AS, *et al.* Critically Ill Patients With Severe Acute Respiratory Syndrome. *JAMA* 2003; 290: 367-373.

[21] Abe M HT, Okada K, Kaizu K, Matsumoto K. Clinical study of influenza-associated rhabdomyolysis with acute renal failure. *Clin. Nephrol.* 2006; 66: 166-170.

[22] Abe M KK, Matsumoto K. Clinical evaluation of pneumonia-associated rhabdomyolysis with acute renal failure. . *Ther. Apher. Dial.* 2008; 12: 171-175.

[23] Ayala E, Kagawa FT, Wehner JH, Tam J, *et al.* Rhabdomyolysis Associated With 2009 Influenza A(H1N1). *JAMA* 2009; 302: 1863-1864.

[24] Gilbertson DT, Ebben JP, Foley RN, Weinhandl ED, *et al.* Hemoglobin Level Variability: Associations with Mortality. *Clin. J. Am. Soc. Nephrol.* 2008; 3: 133-138.

[25] Breen D B, D. Acute renal failure as part of multiple organ failure: The slippery slope of critical illness. *Kidney international* 1998; 53: 25-33.

[26] Chih-Cheng L, Cheng-Yi W, Hen IL. Rhabdomyolysis and Acute Kidney Injury Associated With 2009 Pandemic Influenza A(H1N1). *American journal of kidney diseases : the official journal of the National Kidney Foundation* 55: 615.

[27] Armstrong CL MA, Hsu KC, Gamboa ET. susceptibility of human skeletal muscle culture to influenza virus infection: Cytopathology and immunofluorescence. *J. Neurol. Sci.* 1978; 35: 43-57.

[28] Gu J GE, Zhang B, Zheng J, Gao Z, Zhong Y. Multiple organ infection and the pathogenesis of SARS. *JEM* 2005; 202: 415-424.

[29] Kuiper J GJ, Slutsky A, Plotz F. Mechanical ventilation and acute renal failure. *Crit. Care Med.* 2005; 33: 1408-1415.

[30] Wilson CB SR. Goodpasture's syndrome associated with influenza A2 virus infection. *Ann. Intern Med* 1972; 76: 91-94.

[31] Hauser AB, Stinghen AEM, Kato S, Bucharles S, *et al.* Characteristics and Causes of Immune Dysfunction Related to Uremia and Dialysis. *Perit. Dial. Int.* 2008; 28: S183-187.

[32] Antonen JA HP, Pyhala R, Saha HH, Ala-Houhala IO, Pasternack AI. Adequate seroresponse to influenza vaccination in dialysis patients. *Nephron* 2000; 86: 56-61.

[33] Antonen JA, Pyhala R, Hannula PM, Ala-Houhala IO, *et al.* Influenza vaccination of dialysis patients: cross-reactivity of induced haemagglutination-inhibiting antibodies to H3N2 subtype antigenic variants is comparable with the response of naturally infected young healthy adults. *Nephrol. Dial. Transplant.* 2003; 18: 777-781.

[34] Dharan NJ, Gubareva LV, Meyer JJ, Okomo-Adhiambo M, *et al.* Infections With Oseltamivir-Resistant Influenza A(H1N1) Virus in the United States. *JAMA* 2009; 301: 1034-1041.

[35] Robson R BA, Lynn K, Brewster M, Ward P. The pharmacokinetics and tolerability of oseltamivir suspension in patients on haemodialysis and continuous ambulatory peritoneal dialysis. . *Nephrol. Dial. Transplant.* 2006; 21: 2556-2562.

[36] Marcelli D, Marelli C, Richards N. Influenza A(H1N1)v pandemic in the dialysis population: first wave results from an international survey. *Nephrol. Dial. Transplant.* 2009: gfp557.

[37] Wiebe C RM, Komenda P, Bueti J, Rigatto C, Sood MM. Atypical clinical presentation, course dialysis population: first wave results from an international survey. *Nephrol Dial Transplant* 2009: gfp557.and outcome of H1N1 Influenza A infection in a dialysis patient. *The Lancet* 2009 374: 1300.

In: Acute Kidney Injury: Causes, Diagnosis and Treatments   ISBN: 978-1-61209-790-9
Editor: Jonathan D. Mendoza pp. 111-140   © 2011 Nova Science Publishers, Inc.

Chapter VIII

Biomarkers in Acute Kidney Injury[*]

*Michael A. Ferguson[1†], Vishal S. Vaidya[2] and
Joseph V. Bonventre[3]*
[1]Division of Nephrology, Children's Hospital Boston
Hunnewell 319, Boston, MA 02115, USA
[2]Brigham and Women's Hospital, Harvard Medical School, Renal Division
Harvard Institutes of Medicine, Room 550
4 Blackfan Circle, Boston, MA 02115, USA
[3]Renal Division, Brigham and Women's Hospital, Robert H. Ebert Professor of Medicine
and Health Science and Technology, Harvard Medical School, MIT
Harvard Institutes of Medicine,
Room 576, 4 Blackfan Circle, Boston, MA 02115, USA

Abstract

Acute kidney injury (AKI) is a common condition with significant associated morbidity and mortality. Although impressive progress has been made in the understanding of the molecular and biochemical mechanisms of kidney injury as well as in the clinical care of patients with AKI, outcomes have remained disturbingly static over the last 40 – 50 years. Reliance on current measures of renal dysfunction, such as serum creatinine and blood urea nitrogen, has contributed to the slow translation of basic science discovery to therapeutically effective approaches in clinical practice. Insensitivity of commonly used biomarkers of renal dysfunction not only prevents timely diagnosis and estimation of injury severity, but also delays administration of putative therapeutic agents. A number of serum and urinary proteins have been identified that may herald AKI prior to a rise in serum creatinine. Further characterization of these candidate

---

[*] A version of this chapter was also published in *Biomarkers of Renal Disease,* edited by Mitchell H. Rosner and Mark Osuka, published by Nova Science Publishers, Inc. It was submitted for appropriate modifications in an effort to encourage wider dissemination of research.
[†] Tel: 617-355-6129 ; E-mail: michael.ferguson@childrens.harvard.edu.

biomarkers will clarify their utility and define new diagnostic and prognostic paradigms for AKI, facilitate clinical trials and lead to novel effective therapies. Thus, we are positioned to soon have clinically useful biomarkers which, either alone or in combination, will facilitate earlier diagnosis, earlier targeted intervention, and improved outcomes.

Introduction

Acute renal failure (ARF) has been classically defined as an abrupt and sustained decrease in renal function, resulting in decreased excretion of nitrogenous waste products, as well as disturbed fluid, electrolyte, and acid-base homeostasis. Over the last several decades, numerous advances have been made in the understanding of the pathophysiologic mechanisms implicated in ARF as well as the compensatory repair mechanisms involved in renal recovery from acute injury (Figure 1). It is now well established that a number of pathophysiological mechanisms can contribute to ARF, including alterations in renal perfusion resulting from loss of renal blood flow autoregulation and increased renal vasoconstriction; tubular dysfunction resulting from structural changes, metabolic alterations, loss of cell polarity, cell death and abnormalities of tubuloglomerular balance; as well as a pro-inflammatory milieu resulting from hypoxia/ischemia [1, 2]. In addition, the sequential process of epithelial cell dedifferentiation, proliferation, and eventual redifferentiation in the restoration of the functional integrity of the nephron during recovery has been well described [3, 4]. Clinically, there have been important advances in supportive dialytic technology include the development of biocompatible dialysis membranes, which are associated with reduced complement and granulocyte activation, as well as the development and refinement of continuous renal replacement modalities, which allow for ultrafiltration and solute clearance with less associated hemodynamic compromise [5]. Improvements in the general care and monitoring of patients in the critical care setting are evidenced by improved reported outcomes in patients with sepsis [6], acute lung injury [7, 8], and acute myocardial injury [9]. Despite these advances and the large amount insight into pathophysiology in animal studies, notable improvements in the therapeutics of ARF have been few.

Recent epidemiologic data suggest that the progress observed in the understanding of the pathophysiology of ARF and in the clinical care of patients with ARF have failed to yield commensurate improvements in clinical outcomes. In the adult population, ARF has been reported to complicate 1 − 7% [10-15] of all hospital admissions and 1 − 25% of intensive care unit (ICU) admissions [16, 17]. Over the last 50 years, mortality rates for ARF occurring in the intensive care unit have remained essentially unchanged at approximately 50 − 70% [18]. A recent large international study of the epidemiology and outcome of ARF in critically ill adult patients reported an overall in-hospital mortality rate of 60% [19]. Of those who survived to hospital discharge, 13% remained dialysis dependent. In a smaller retrospective study of 267 adult ARF survivors requiring acute renal replacement therapy, renal insufficiency persisted in 41% and overall 5-year survival post-discharge was 50% [13]. Epidemiologic data for ARF in the pediatric population, although notably sparse, reflects similar trends. One recent retrospective review reported an in-hospital mortality rate of 30% [20], essentially unchanged from that reported 30 years ago [21]. Of those patients requiring intensive care unit admission and renal replacement therapy, mortality rates were 40% and

44% respectively [20]. Longitudinal follow-up of survivors to hospital discharge revealed a 3-5 year survival rate of 80%. Of those assessed for long-term sequelae at 3-5 years, 59% (17/29) exhibited at least one sign of chronic kidney disease including microalbuminuria, hyperfiltration, decreased glomerular filtration rate (GFR), and/or hypertension [22].

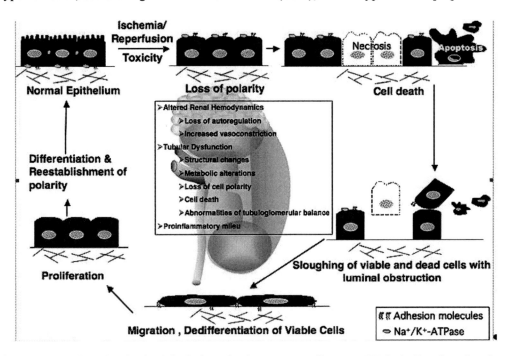

Figure 1. A number of pathophysiological mechanisms can contribute to AKI, including alterations in renal perfusion resulting from loss of autoregulation and increased renal vasoconstriction; tubular dysfunction resulting from structural changes, metabolic alterations, loss of cell polarity, cell death and abnormalities of tubuloglomerular balance; as well as a pro-inflammatory milieu resulting from hypoxia/ischemia. Subsequent restoration of the functional integrity of the nephron involves the ordered process of epithelial cell dedifferentiation, proliferation, and eventual redifferentiation. (Adapted from Vaidya, Ferguson, and Bonventre, Annual Reviews of Pharmacology and Toxicology, 2007).

Over the last 10 years, in response to such disturbingly static outcome data, increased attention has been focused on identifying and addressing impediments to progress in ARF research. In 2000, the Acute Dialysis Quality Initiative (ADQI) was formed with the goal of establishing an evidence-based appraisal and set of consensus recommendations to standardize care and direct further research in the field of ARF [23]. One problem area identified was the relative lack of consensus regarding criteria used to define ARF. Historically, authors have used different measures to assess renal function as well as varied criteria as cut-offs to guide diagnosis. It is estimated that more than 30 different definitions of ARF exist in the published literature [24], ranging from severe (ARF requiring dialysis) to mild (modest observable increases in serum creatinine) [9]. As a result of the disparate clinical and physiologic endpoints used to guide investigation, epidemiologic studies as well as trials of prevention and intervention are often not comparable. As part of the ADQI 2nd International Consensus Conference, the RIFLE classification scheme (Risk of kidney dysfunction; Injury to the kidney; Failure of kidney function; Loss of kidney function; and End stage kidney disease) was derived to provide standardized criteria for defining ARF with the goal of facilitating comparison of outcomes across studies, development of prognostic scoring systems, interpretation of therapeutic intervention strategies, and design of multicenter studies [25]. This work ultimately led to the introduction of the term "acute kidney injury" (AKI) as the preferred nomenclature for the clinical disorder formally called ARF (from this point on AKI will be used to describe the clinical condition formally referred to as ARF). This transition served to emphasize the notion that the spectrum of disease is much broader than that subset of patients who experience failure requiring dialysis support [26]. This new nomenclature underscores the fact that kidney injury exists along a continuum: the more severe the injury, the more likely the overall outcome will be unfavorable.

More recently, the Acute Kidney Injury Network (AKIN) was formed in an effort to facilitate improved care of patients with or at risk for AKI. In recognition of increasing data suggesting that even small changes in serum creatinine are associated with poorer outcome as measured by mortality [27, 28], the AKIN committee proposed uniform standards for defining, diagnosing, and classifying AKI. This group defined AKI as "functional or structural abnormalities or markers of kidney damage including abnormalities in blood, urine, or tissues tests or imaging studies present for less than three months [29]." The committee set diagnostic criteria for AKI as "an abrupt (within 48 hours) reduction in kidney function currently defined as an absolute increase in serum creatinine of either ≥ 0.3 mg/dl or a percentage increase of $\geq 50\%$ or a documented reduction in urine output (documented oliguria of < 0.5 ml/kg/h for > 6 hours [29]." The oliguria criteria assume adequate hydration, although adequate hydration is not well defined. Appropriate modifications to the RIFLE criteria were made to modify the Risk criteria to include an absolute increase in serum creatinine ≥ 0.3 mg/dl (Table 1). Of note, a group of pediatric nephrologists and intensivists have proposed and validated modifications to existing RIFLE criteria for use in pediatric patients with or at risk for AKI (Table 2) [30].

Although clear progress has been made in formulating a consensus definition, diagnostic criteria, and classification scheme for AKI, it is notable that all are heavily dependent on changes in serum creatinine as a marker of injury. Unfortunately, creatinine is a suboptimal marker following injury; levels are often not reflective of glomerular filtration rate (GFR) due to a number of renal and non-renal influences [31]. In the setting of AKI, the dynamic relationship between serum creatinine and GFR inhibits the ability to accurately estimate timing of injury and severity of dysfunction following injury [32]. A sudden fall in GFR to a constant low level causes a gradual increase in serum creatinine until a new steady state between generation and excretion is achieved. The rate of rise following AKI is dependent on many factors including the new GFR, rate of tubular secretion, rate of generation, and volume of distribution [31, 32]. As a result, large changes in GFR may be associate with relatively small changes in serum creatinine in the first $24 - 48$ hours following AKI, resulting not only in delayed diagnosis and intervention, but also in underestimation of the degree of injury [31]. In addition, there is considerable variability among patients in the correlation between serum creatinine and baseline GFR, in the magnitude of functional renal reserve, and in creatinine synthesis rates. As a result, a renal injury of comparable magnitude may result in disparate alterations in creatinine concentration in different individuals [25].

The insensitivity and non-specificity of serum creatinine as well other traditionally used markers of renal injury, including blood urea nitrogen, urine sediment, and urinary indices (fractional excretion of sodium, urine osmolality, etc.), have been major obstacles in developing strategies to ameliorate AKI. Results from interventional trials suggesting inefficacy of putative therapies of AKI are by definition confounded by delayed diagnosis and treatment. This paradigm is analogous to the initiation of therapy in patients with myocardial infarction or stroke 48 hours after the onset of ischemia [33].

Table 1. Proposed classification scheme for acute kidney injury (AKI)
(Modified RIFLE Criteria)*

Stage	Creatinine criteria	Urine output criteria
1 (Risk)	Increased SCr of $\geq$ 0.3 mg/dl or increase to $\geq$ 150 – 200% of baseline	UO < 0.5 ml/kg/h for > 6 h
2 (Injury)	Increased SCr to > 200 – 300% of baseline	UO < 0.5 ml/kg/h for > 12 h
3 (Failure)	Increased SCr to > 300% of baseline or SCr $\geq$ 4 mg/dl (acute rise $\geq$ 0.5 mg/dl)	UO < 0.3 ml/kg/h x 24 h or anuria x 12 h
Stages eliminated from original RIFLE criteria		
Loss	Persistent ARF = complete loss of kidney function > 4 weeks	
ESKD	End stage kidney disease (> 3 months)	

ARF: Acute renal failure; ESKD: End stage kidney disease;
RIFLE: Risk of renal dysfunction; Injury to the kidney; Failure of kidney function; Loss of kidney function; End stage kidney disease; SCr: Serum creatinine; UO: Urine output.
*Adapted from ML, Kellum JA, Shah S, Molitoris BA, Ronco C, Warnock D, Levin A. 2006. AKIN: Acute Kidney Injury Network: report of an initiative. In: AKIN Summit 2005. AKIN Committee, Amsterdam, The Netherlands.

Table 2. Proposed classification scheme for pediatric acute kidney injury (AKI)
(Pediatric Modified RIFLE Criteria)*

	Creatinine criteria	Urine output criteria
Risk	eCCl decrease by 25%	UO < 0.5 ml/kg/h for > 8 h
Injury	eCCL decrease by 50%	UO < 0.5 ml/kg/h for > 16 h
Failure	eCCl decrease by 75% *or* eCCl < 35 ml/min/1.73m^2	UO < 0.3 ml/kg/h x 24 h or anuria x 12 h
Loss	Persistent failure > 4 weeks	
End stage	End stage renal disease (> 3 months)	

eCCl: Estimated creatinine clearance.
RIFLE: Risk of renal dysfunction; Injury to the kidney; Failure of kidney function; Loss of kidney function; End stage kidney disease.
UO: Urine output.
* Adapted from Akcan-Arikan A, Zapitelli M, Loftus L , Washburn K, Jefferson LS, Goldstein SL. 2007. Modified RIFLE criteria in critically ill children with acute kidney injury. *Kidney Int.* 71:1028-1035.

Intensive investigative efforts have led to the identification and evaluation of many urinary and serum proteins as potential biomarkers of AKI [33, 34]. In general, serum markers of nephron damage may be of relatively limited utility if they are sensitive to modification by any factor that may alter renal perfusion with subsequent changes in filtration that may or may not be associated with injury (e.g. volume depletion, hemorrhage, or decreased effective intravascular volume in congestive heart failure or cirrhosis). In addition, when elevated serum levels are observed in the setting of a primary renal insult, serum biomarkers have limited utility in determining the location or mechanism of injury unless they are known to only derive from the kidney [35]. As a result, much of the focus in new biomarker development has focused on the examination of urine proteins and metabolites. Studies have yielded many promising urinary candidates for the early detection of AKI and further characterization is anticipated to aid in earlier diagnosis, identification of mechanism of injury, and assessment of site and severity of injury. Hopefully these biomarkers, either alone or in combination, will prove to be useful in guiding targeted intervention and monitoring of disease progression and resolution. The large majority of existing studies have focused on animal models and adult patients at risk for or with established AKI. It should be emphasized, however, that pediatric patients represent an important subpopulation for study as they generally lack co-morbidities such as hypertension, atherosclerosis, and diabetes that affect kidney structure and function and as a result may prove to have very different biomarker profiles than adults [36].

Existing biomarkers of AKI may be broadly classified into two categories: 1) proteins with enzymatic activity that are leaked into the urine following injury; and 2) urinary proteins without known enzymatic activity that are either upregulated or specifically released into the urine in the setting of cellular injury. Table 3 provides a general overview of these candidate biomarkers with appropriate references for further review. Detailed information regarding the most promising biomarkers and a description of knowledge garnered to date follows.

Urinary Proteins with Enzymatic Activity

Urinary enzymes have been extensively studied in a number of pathologic conditions predisposing to renal injury, including nephrotoxin exposure, diabetic nephropathy, hypertension, renal ischemia, renal transplantation, glomerulopathies and the use of shock-wave lithotripsy in the treatment of urinary tract calculi. In the setting of acute or chronic damage, enzymes physiologically present in the tubular epithelium may be released into the urine secondary to leakage from damaged cells or secondary to intensified enzyme induction during the repair and regeneration process[35, 37]. Urinary enzymes have been found to be sensitive biomarkers of AKI that result in dose-dependent increases in urinary enzymatic activity correlated to the degree of tissue damage present [35, 38].

In addition, preclinical and clinical studies have lead to extensive knowledge regarding segmental nephron distribution and cellular ultrastructural (brush border, lysosome, or cytoplasm) location of tubular enzymes.

As a result, enzyme detection in the urine potentially provides valuable information not only pertinent to the site of tubular injury (proximal vs. distal tubule) but also the severity of injury. As a general rule, brush border enzymuria is indicative of a less severe injury than lysosomal or cytosolic enzymuria [35, 37, 38]. It should be noted, however, that despite the theoretical advantage of identifying the primary site of nephron injury, thus far enzymatic markers have not proven effective in differentiating between predominate proximal or distal tubular involvement [37].

Measurement of some urinary enzymes is readily performed with existing colorimetric assays and commercially available ELISA kits. Although these quantification methods have been extensively validated and are highly reproducible, they do not lend themselves to the high-throughput analysis preferable when analyzing large numbers of samples over extended time courses [33].

Table 3. Biomarkers of Acute Kidney Injury

Urinary Proteins with Enzymatic Activity	Comments	Detection	References
Alanine aminopeptidase	1) Proximal tubule brush border enzyme 2) Instability may limit clinical utility	Colorimetry	[39, 135-137]
Alkaline phosphatase	1) Proximal tubule brush border enzyme. Human intestinal alkaline phosphatase is specific for proximal tubular S3 segment; human tissue non-specific alkaline phosphatase is specific for S1 and S2 segments. 2) Levels may not correlate with extent of functional injury 3) Instability may limit clinical utility	Colorimetry	[38, 73, 138, 139]
α-Glutathione-S-transferase	1) Proximal tubule cytosolic enzyme 2) Requires stabilization buffer for specimen storage and processing	ELISA	[33, 38, 140-142]
π-Glutathione-S-transferase	1) Distal tubule brush border enzyme 2) Requires stabilization buffer for specimen storage and processing	ELISA	[38, 140, 141]
γ-Glutamyl transpeptidase	1) Proximal tubule brush border enzyme 2)Instability requires samples to be analyzed quickly after collection, limiting clinical utility	Colorimetry	[35, 38, 136, 143]
N-acetyl-β-D-glucosaminidase	1) Proximal tubule lysosomal enzyme 2) More stable than other urinary enzymes 3) Extensive clinical data in a variety of conditions (nephrotoxicant exposure, cardiopulmonary bypass, delayed renal allograft function, etc.) 4) Endogenous urea may inhibit activity	Colorimetry	[33, 35, 37-39, 45]
Filtered low-molecular weight proteins			
α1-microglobulin	1) Synthesized by the liver 2) Filtered by the glomerulus and reabsorbed by proximal tubule cells 3) Early marker of tubular dysfunction; high levels may predict poorer outcome 4) Stable across physiologic urinary pH	ELISA; nephelometry	[35, 54-56]
β2-microglobulin	1) Light chain of the MHC I molecule expressed on the cell surface of all nucleated cells 2) Monomeric form is filtered by the glomerulus and reabsorbed by the proximal tubule cells 3) Early marker of tubular dysfunction in a variety of conditions 4) Instability in acidic urine limits clinical utility	ELISA; nephelometry	[48-51, 53]

Table 3. (Continued)

Urinary Antigens	Comments	Detection	References
Cystatin-C	1) Important extracellular inhibitor of cysteine proteases 2) Filtered by the glomerulus and reabsorbed by proximal tubule cells 3) Elevated urinary levels reflect tubular dysfunction; high levels may predict poorer outcome	ELISA; nephelometry	[54, 60-62]
Retinol binding protein	1) Synthesized by liver, involved in vitamin A transport 2) Filtered by glomerulus and reabsorbed by proximal tubule cells 3) Early marker of tubular dysfunction 4) Increased stability in acidic urine when compared to β_2-microglobulin	ELISA; nephelometry	[48, 58, 59]
Heart-type fatty acid binding protein	1) Expressed in distal tubule epithelial cells 2) Functions in intracellular fatty acid transport to sites of β-oxidation 3) May serve as useful marker in assessment of non-heart beating donor organs for kidney transplantation	ELISA	[94, 97, 99, 100]
Liver-type fatty acid binding protein	1) Expressed in proximal tubule epithelial cells 2) Important functions include intracellular fatty acid transport and possible sequestration of reactive fatty acid oxidation products 3) Current evidence suggests clinical utility as a biomarker in CKD and diabetic nephropathy 4) Additional studies necessary to determine utility in setting of AKI	ELISA	[94, 96, 98, 102, 104, 105, 107, 107a, 107b, 144]
Interleukin-18	1) Cytokine with broad immunomodulatory properties, particularly in setting of ischemic injury 2) Constitutively expressed in distal tubules; strong immunoreactivity in proximal tubules with transplant rejection 3) Elevated urinary levels found to be early marker of AKI and independent predictor of mortality in critically ill patients	ELISA; Luminex	[86, 88-93]
Kidney Injury Molecule-1	1) Type-1 cell membrane glycoprotein upregulated in dedifferentiated proximal tubule epithelial cells 2) Protein ectodomain shed into urine following acute injury 3) Elevated urinary levels found to be highly sensitive and specific for AKI	ELISA; Luminex	[64, 69, 71-73]

Urinary Antigens (cont.)	Comments	Detection	References
Neutrophil gelatinase-associated lipocalin	1) Initially identified bound to gelatinase in specific granules of the, but also may be induced in epithelial cells in the setting of inflammation or malignancy 2) Expression upregulated in distal tubule cells following ischemic renal injury 3) Uptake of filtered molecule by the proximal tubule is reduced following injury 4) Found to be an early indicator of AKI following cardiopulmonary bypass 5) Specificity for AKI in setting of sepsis, pyuria needs to be further established	ELISA	[74, 76, 77, 80, 81, 145, 146]
Exosome Associated Proteins Exosomal fetuin-A	1) Acute phase protein synthesized in the liver and secreted into the circulation 2) Levels in proximal tubule cell cytoplasm correspond to degree of injury 3) Urinary levels found to be much higher in ICU patients with AKI compared to ICU patients without AKI and healthy volunteers 4) Samples require considerable processing, limiting assay throughput	Immunoblot	[111, 117, 118]
Na+/H+ exchanger isoform 3	1) Most abundant sodium transporter in the renal tubule 2) Urinary levels found to discriminate between prerenal azotemia and AKI in ICU patients 3) Samples require considerable processing, limiting assay throughput	Immunoblot	[112, 116, 117]

N-acetyl-β-glucosaminidase (NAG). NAG, a proximal tubule lysosomal enzyme, has been extensively studied in both the adult and pediatric population and has proven to be a sensitive, persistent, and robust indicator of AKI. Increased NAG levels have been reported with nephrotoxin exposure [35, 37], delayed renal allograft function [39], chronic glomerular disease [40], diabetic nephropathy [41], as well as following cardiopulmonary bypass procedures [42]. Westhuyzen et al. [38] reported that urinary NAG levels (in addition to other tubular enzymes) were highly sensitive in detecting AKI in a population of critically ill adult patients, preceding increases in serum creatinine by 12 hours to 4 days. Chew et al. [43] reported a poorer outcome (death in hospital, requirement for long term renal replacement therapy) in patients with higher urinary NAG levels on admission to a renal care unit, indicating a dose response correlating injury with outcome. The greater the urinary NAG level in patients already diagnosed with AKI by clinical criteria, the greater the incidence of the combined end point of dialysis or death [44]. However, urinary NAG activity has been found to be inhibited by endogenous urea [45] as well as a number of nephotoxins and heavy metals [33]. In addition, given the various conditions that have been associated with increased NAG excretion, non-specificity for AKI may limit its use as a biomarker.

Other enzymatic markers. A number of important disadvantages have been noted with respect to the use of enzymuria in the setting AKI. Although highly sensitive for renal injury, the utility of urinary enzymes has been clouded by the low threshold for release in response to physiologic conditions that may not precede clinically significant AKI [37]. Perhaps more important from a practical viewpoint is the instability of many urinary enzymes and the specific processing necessary to ensure integrity in samples [35]. For example, the brush border enzymes alanine aminopeptidase (AA), alkaline phosphatase (AP), and γ-glutamyl transpeptidase (γ-GT) are stable for only 4 hours after urine collection and samples require gel filtration to eliminate interfering substances [33]. Alpha-glutathione-S-transferase (α-GST) and π-glutathione-S-transferase (π-GST), cytosolic enzymes that have been found to be rapidly released in the urine following proximal and distal tubular injury respectively, [46] require a specific stabilization buffer to ensure appropriate quantification.

In general, the utility of urinary enzyme excretion as diagnostic or predictive biomarkers for AKI remains an area that warrants additional investigation. Further characterization is needed to determine threshold levels indicative of clinically significant injury and if the theoretic advantage of identifying the primary site of tubule injury will translate to a clinically important advantage by guiding intervention. In addition, it will be important to develop user friendly approaches to sample preservation and quantification to allow for high throughput processing of samples necessary for large scale studies and clinical assessment.

Other Urinary Antigens

A number of other urinary antigens have been evaluated as potential biomarkers of AKI. Filtered low molecular weight proteins, including $α_1$-microglobulin, $β_1$-microglobulin, cystatin C, and retinol binding protein (RBP) have been studied extensively over the last 2 decades. More recently, proteomic and genomic screening modalities have identified numerous tubular proteins that are markedly upregulated and/or excreted in the setting of renal injury. These novel proteins have generated significant excitement in the research community not only as candidate biomarkers of AKI, but also as molecules that may play critical roles in the regulation of cell dedifferentiation, migration, and proliferation in response to injury. It is anticipated that further investigative efforts will not only define the utility of these proteins as biomarkers, but also enhance our understanding of the pathophysiology of AKI and aid in the development of targeted interventions to ameliorate injury with the ultimate goal of improving outcomes.

Filtered Low-Molecular Weight Proteins

The finding of elevated levels of filtered low-molecular weight proteins (β_2-microglobulin, α_1-microglobulin, retinol-binding protein, and cystatin C) in the urine is reflective of a primary defect in proximal tubular uptake, which may occur in the setting of cellular damage or overload of cellular uptake processes. Produced at different non-renal sites, these proteins are freely filtered by the glomerulus and reabsorbed but not secreted by proximal tubular cells. Injury to the proximal tubular epithelium leads to diminished microvillus surface area of the brush border membrane and reduced reabsorptive capacity. The resultant tubular proteinuria has been extensively studied as an index of tubular injury. As a general rule, the utility of low-molecular weight filtered proteins as biomarkers in the setting of AKI is limited by concomitant significant glomerular proteinuria or hyperfiltration, situations where the tubular reabsorptive pathways may be saturated [47]. Furthermore, specificity for acute injury is suboptimal.

Beta$_2$-microglobulin (β_2M). β_2M is an 11.8 kilodalton (kDa) protein that functions as the light chain of the major histocompatibility class (MHC) I molecule, which is expressed on the cell surface of all nucleated cells. β_2M dissociates from the heavy chain in the setting of cellular turnover and enters the circulation as a monomer [48]. β_2M is typically filtered by the glomerulus and almost entirely reabsorbed and catabolized by the proximal tubular cells [49], a process that may be impeded with AKI. Increased urinary β_2M excretion has been observed to be an early marker of tubular injury in a number of settings including nephrotoxin exposure [50], cardiac surgery [51, 52], and renal transplantation [53]. In these settings, rises in β_2M precede rises in serum creatinine by as much as 4 – 5 days [48]. Unfortunately, the utility of β_2M as a biomarker has been limited by its instability in the urine, with rapid degradation observed at room temperature and in urine with a pH less than 6.0. Schaub et al. [53] recently identified cleaved urinary β_2M as a potential biomarker of tubular injury in renal allografts; however, assays for protein quantification have not been developed. It should also be noted that although β_2M may serve as an early biomarker for AKI, it has been found to be poorly predictive of severe injury requiring renal replacement therapy (RRT) [54].

Alpha$_1$-microglobulin (α_1M). α_1M is a 27 – 33 kDa protein synthesized by the liver with approximately half of the circulating protein complexed to IgA. The free form is readily filtered by the glomerulus and reabsorbed by proximal tubule cells. Unlike β_2M, urinary α_1M is stable over the range of pH found in routine clinical practice [35, 55], making it a preferred marker of tubular proteinuria in human bioassays. It has been found to be a sensitive biomarker for proximal tubular dysfunction even in the early phase of injury when no histologic damage is observable [56]. In a heterogeneous population of patients with non-oliguric AKI, Herget-Rosenthal et al. reported α_1M to be an early indicator of unfavorable outcome (requirement for RRT) [54]. In addition, urinary α_1M has been proposed to be a useful marker of tubular dysfunction even in low gestational age preterm infants, a population at high risk for AKI [57].

Retinol binding protein (RBP). RBP is a 21 kDa protein that is hepatically synthesized and responsible for transporting vitamin A from the liver to other tissues. It is freely filtered by the glomerulus and subsequently reabsorbed and catabolized by the proximal tubule. Bernard et al. [58] monitored patients with AKI from various etiologies and found urinary RBP to be a highly sensitive indicator of renal tubule dysfunction, preceding urinary NAG elevation. They reported RBP and β_2M levels to be highly correlated when urinary pH > 6.0 with progressively increasing RBP/β_2M ratios as urinary pH declined, reflecting RBPs stability in acidic urine when compared to the instability of β_2M [58]. In addition, Roberts et al. [59] reported that increased RBP levels during the first two days of life were predictive of clinically significant AKI in infants following birth asphyxia, a setting where interpretation of serum creatinine is particularly problematic as it reflects maternal serum concentration to a significant extent. It should be noted that serum RBP levels are depressed in vitamin A deficiency and urinary levels may theoretically yield a false negative result in this setting [48].

Cystatin C. Cystatin-C (Cys-C) is a 13 kDa protein that is believed to be one of the most important extracellular inhibitors of cysteine proteases. Serum concentrations appear to be independent of sex, age, and muscle mass. Cys-C is freely filtered by the glomerulus, reabsorbed and catabolized, but not secreted by the tubules. Over the last decade, serum Cys-C has been extensively studied and found to be a sensitive serum marker of GFR and a stronger predictor of risk of death and cardiovascular events in older patients than serum creatinine [60]. Urinary Cys-C levels have been found to be elevated in individuals with known tubular dysfunction [61, 62]. In addition, Herget-Rosenthal et al. reported that elevated urinary Cys-C levels were highly predictive of poor outcome (requirement for RRT) in a heterogeneous group of patients with initially non-oliguric AKI [54]. There are no published reports of the utility of urinary Cys-C in the setting of pediatric AKI; however, an interesting study revealed that fetal urinary Cys-C levels were predictive of post-natal renal dysfunction in the setting of bilateral uropathies [63].

Kidney Injury Molecule-1 (KIM-1)

KIM-1 is a type I cell membrane glycoprotein containing a unique six-cysteine immunoglobulin-like domain and a mucin domain in its extracellular portion [64]. Rat and human cDNAs encoding KIM-1 (Kim-1 in the rat) were initially identified by our group using representational difference analysis, a polymerase-chain reaction-based cDNA subtraction analysis designed to identify genes with differential expression between normal and regenerating kidneys following ischemia/reperfusion (I/R) injury [64]. Kim-1 was subsequently found to be expressed at low to undetectable levels in the normal adult rat kidney but dramatically upregulated in the post-ischemic kidney. In-situ hybridization and immunohistochemistry studies demonstrated that Kim-1 mRNA and protein are expressed in proximal tubule epithelial cells in damaged regions. Kim-1 immunoreactivity was co-localized with the dedifferentiation protein vimentin and the proliferation marker BrdU [64]. Independently, a large pharmaceutical consortium, using an unbiased genomic approach, determined that Kim-1 was upregulated more than any other of the 30,000 genes tested in response to the nephrotoxin cisplatin [65]. Thus, structure and expression data suggest that KIM-1 is an epithelial adhesion molecule upregulated in dedifferentiating and regenerating tubule epithelial cells following injury and may play a role in the restoration of morphological integrity of the tubule [64].

Our group later reported that the KIM-1 ectodomain was shed from cells *in vitro* [66] and into the urine *in vivo* in rodents and humans after proximal tubular injury of varying etiology [67-70]. Urinary KIM-1 quantification was initially performed via an enzyme-linked immunosorbent assay (ELISA) and subsequently by a high-throughput microbead based assay that offers increased sensitivity and a greater dynamic range [71, 72]. Urinary KIM-1 has been found to be an early indicator of AKI that compares favorably to a number of conventional biomarkers and tubular enzymes [72, 73]. In the setting of cisplatin exposure as well as renal I/R in rats, Kim-1 was found to have superior sensitivity for detecting AKI, over that seen with serum creatinine and BUN or urinary NAG, glycosuria, and proteinuria [72].

A number of human studies have confirmed the promise of urinary KIM-1 for the diagnosis and prediction of outcome of AKI. Adjusted for age, gender, and length of time delay between insult and sampling, Han et al. reported that a one-unit increase in normalized KIM-1 was associated with a greater than 12-fold increase in the presence of acute tubular necrosis (ATN) [73]. Liangos et al. [73a] demonstrated that elevated urinary KIM-1 and NAG were significantly associated with severity of AKI as determined by the composite endpoint of death or dialysis requirement. Van Timmeren et al. [73b] reported proximal tubule KIM-1 staining in biopsy specimens of 102 patients with AKI from varying etiology to be correlated with tubulo-interstitial fibrosis and inflammation. Furthermore, urinary KIM-1 levels correlated with tissue expression of KIM-1 in a subset of patients who underwent urine collection at the time of biopsy [73b]. In addition, Zhang et al. showed that KIM-1 expression quantified by immunohistochemical staining in renal transplant biopsies sensitively and specifically identified proximal tubule injury and correlated with renal function [73c]. KIM-1 expression was more sensitive than histology for detecting early tubular injury and KIM-1 expression may be indicative of the potential for renal recovery in the setting of injury [73c]. Thus, KIM-1 is a sensitive, specific, and stable biomarker of AKI in both cross-sectional and prospective adult clinical studies.

Neutrophil Gelatinase-Associated Lipocalin (NGAL)

Human NGAL is a 25 kDa protein initially identified bound to gelatinase in specific granules of the neutrophil. NGAL is synthesized during a narrow window of granulocyte maturation in the bone marrow [74], but also may be induced in epithelial cells in the setting of inflammation or malignancy [75]. Cowland and Borregaard demonstrated varying degrees of NGAL gene expression in a number of other human tissues including the uterus, prostate, salivary gland, lung, trachea, stomach, colon and kidney [76]. Using cDNA microarray screening techniques, Devarajan and colleagues identified NGAL as one of seven genes whose expression was upregulated > 10-fold within the first few hours after ischemic renal injury in a mouse model [77]. Immunohisotochemistry studies demonstrated minimal NGAL expression in control mouse kidneys, but marked increase in proximal tubules within 3 hours of ischemia [77]. Examination of serial kidney sections revealed significant colocalization of NGAL and the proliferative marker PCNA [77]. In addition, it has been reported that NGAL induces the conversion of rat kidney progenitors into tubules and epithelia [78]. As a result, it has been hypothesized that NGAL may play a role in the induction of tubular re-epithelialization in the setting of AKI.

Subsequent studies suggest that NGAL accumulates in a renal as well as a systemic pool in the setting of AKI [78a, 78b]. There is rapid and robust upregulation of NGAL mRNA in the thick ascending limb and collecting ducts with associated synthesis of NGAL in the distal nephron in AKI (the renal pool) [78a, 78b]. In addition, AKI results in increased mRNA expression in other organs, including the liver and lung, with subsequent release into the circulation (the systemic pool) [78a, 78b]. The renal pool is believed to represent the major contributor to urinary NGAL; however, insufficient tubular reabsorption of filtered NGAL from the systemic pool should contribute to urinary NGAL levels as well.

Increased NGAL levels were readily detected in the urine of rodents following I/R injury and after cisplatin exposure, preceding changes in serum creatinine as well as the appearance of urinary β_2M and NAG [77, 79]. As a result, NGAL has generated much interest as a sensitive early biomarker for diagnosing AKI. A prospective study of pediatric patients undergoing cardiopulmonary bypass for cardiac corrective surgery found urinary NGAL to be a powerful early marker of AKI, preceding any increase in serum creatinine by $1 - 3$ days [80]. A similar study of adult patients showed urinary NGAL levels at 1, 3, and 18 hours after cardiac surgery to be significantly higher in patients who went on to develop clinically significant AKI [81]. A retrospective analysis of urine samples from patients with diarrhea-associated hemolytic uremic syndrome revealed that normal urinary NGAL excretion during the early stages of hospitalization had a high negative predictive value of the need for dialysis; however, high urinary NGAL levels were not a reliable predictor of need for dialysis [82]. Systemic NGAL levels are known to rise in the setting of a number of inflammatory and infective conditions with and without concomitant kidney injury [83, 84, 84a, 84b]. Further studies are required to determine specificity of urinary NGAL for AKI in the setting of sepsis, a condition frequently associated with clinically significant renal injury.

Interleukin-18 (IL-18)

IL-18, formerly known as interferon-γ-inducing factor, is produced as a 24 kDa inactive precursor that is cleaved by caspase-1 to generate its mature, biologically active form [85-87]. IL-18 has been found to have broad immunomodulatory properties and appears to play a critical role in host defense against a number of infections [86]. In addition, IL-18 activity has been described in a number of inflammatory diseases across a broad range of tissues, including inflammatory arthritis, multiple sclerosis, inflammatory bowel disease, chronic hepatitis, systemic lupus erythematosis, and psoriasis [86]. There are reports indicating that IL-18 is an important mediator in tissue I/R injury. In an I/R model of human myocardium, diminished IL-18 activity through selective caspase-1 inhibition was found to protect against injury and resulted in significant preservation of myocardial contractile force [88]. In preclinical studies, caspase-1 inhibition or the administration of IL-18-neutralizing serum was found to protect against ischemic AKI in mice [89, 90].

Parikh et al. reported increased levels of IL-18 in patients with AKI of varying etiology, especially those with delayed renal allograft function and ischemic ATN [91]. Following transplantation, a rapid decline in urinary IL-18 levels was predictive of a steeper decline in serum creatinine concentrations postoperative days 0 – 4 [91]. Immunohistochemical staining of renal transplant protocol biopsies revealed constitutive IL-18 expression in the distal tubular epithelium. There was strong positive immunoreactivity in the proximal tubules of patients with acute rejection. There was also strong immunoreactivity in infiltrating leukocytes, and endothelium, suggesting upregulation in the setting of immunopathological reactions [92]. In a study of critically ill adult patients with acute respiratory distress syndrome (ARDS), increased urinary IL-18 was found to be an early marker of AKI, preceding changes in serum creatinine by 1 – 2 days, and was an independent predictor of death [93]. To date, the utility of urinary IL-18 as a biomarker of AKI has not been established in the pediatric population.

Fatty Acid Binding Protein (FABP)

The fatty acid binding proteins (FAPB) are small cytoplasmic proteins abundantly expressed in tissues with an active fatty acid binding metabolism. Nine different types have been identified with each named for the initial site of identification [94]. The primary function of FABP is the facilitation of long-chain free fatty-acid transport from the plasma membrane to sites for oxidation (mitochondria, peroxisomes) [94, 95]. Increased levels of cystosolic free fatty acids with attendant increased FABP expression may be seen in response to a variety of pathophysiologic tubular stresses [94]. There is evidence that FABP may serve as an endogenous antioxidant, not only binding polyunsaturated fatty acids and protecting them from oxidation but also binding fatty acid oxidation products, thereby limiting the toxic effects of oxidative intermediates on cellular membranes [96]. Two types of FABP have been identified in the human kidney, liver-type FABP (L-FABP) in the proximal tubule and heart-type FABP (H-FABP) in the distal tubule [97, 98].

H-FABP levels have been found to be a sensitive marker for nephrotoxin induced kidney injury in rats [94]. In addition, H-FABP has been studied as a marker of tissue damage resulting from pre-transplantation machine perfusion in the preparation of non-heart beating donor (NHBD) organs for kidney transplantation. Higher levels of H-FABP, as well as other biomarkers, in kidney perfusates were determined to be useful adjuncts to routine indicators (donor age, donor medical history, macroscopic appearance, warm ischemic time, and ex-vivo perfusion) of suitability of NHBD kidneys for transplantation [94, 99, 100]. Clinical studies into the utility of H-FABP as a urinary biomarker in more conventional models of AKI are lacking.

Urinary L-FABP has been studied extensively in preclinical and clinical models and has been found to be a potential biomarker in a number of pathologic conditions, including chronic kidney disease, diabetic nephropathy, IgA nephropathy, contrast nephropathy, nephrotoxin exposure, and ischemic injury. Using human L-FABP (hL-FABP) chromosomal transgenic mice, it has been demonstrated that protein-overload nephropathy and unilateral ureteral obstruction, two models of renal interstitial injury, are associated with increased expression and urinary excretion of hL-FABP [101, 102]. In both injury models, attenuation of tubulointerstitial damage was observed in the transgenic mice when compared to wild-type mice, supporting the notion that L-FABP plays a protective role in the setting of increased renal tubular stress [101, 102]. In clinical studies, L-FABP has been advocated as a potential biomarker for monitoring progression of CKD. Kamijo et al. reported increasing L-FABP levels with deterioration of renal function in those subjects with non-diabetic CKD [102]. Further studies in type II diabetics have shown an association between the stage of diabetic nephropathy and urinary L-FAPB levels [103] as well as the potential benefit of renin-angiotensin system blockade in this population, reflected in decreased L-FABP excretion [104]. Nakamura et al. have reported that urinary L-FABP may serve as a non-invasive biomarker to discriminate between IgA nephropathy and thin basement membrane disease [105] as well as a potential predictive marker for contrast-induced nephropathy [106]. More recent studies point to utility in more traditional models of AKI. Yamamoto et al. reported urinary L-FABP to be highly correlated with ischemia time as well as length of hospital stay in a cohort of living related kidney transplant recipients [107]. Our recent work found urinary L-FABP levels to be highly sensitive and specific for AKI in a cross-sectional study of adult patients with established AKI from varying etiologies [107a]. In addition, Portilla et al. reported that urinary L-FABP levels were predictive of subsequent AKI within 4 hours after cardiac surgery in a cohort of pediatric patients [107b].

Urinary L-FABP may be non-specific for AKI in the setting of acute liver injury. Although Kamijo et al. reported urinary L-FABP levels in patients with liver disease to be similar to levels in healthy volunteers, it is unclear if these patients suffered from acute or chronic liver injury [102]. This will be important to investigate as AKI and acute liver injury commonly co-occur in the critically ill population.

Exosome Associated Proteins

Quantitating the content of urinary exosomes has recently emerged as an approach meriting further investigation in the discovery and mechanistic description of urinary biomarkers in AKI. Exosomes are created when a segment of the cell membrane invaginates and undergoes endocytosis. This *endosome* is shuttled to a multivesicular body (MVB) where proteins are segregated in the outer membrane and subsequently internalized by membrane invagination, forming *internal vesicles*. Eventually, the outer membrane of the MVB fuses with the apical plasma membrane, releasing its internal vesicles, or *exosomes*, into the urinary space [108]. Urinary exosomes contain both membrane and cytosolic proteins that may serve as biomarkers for a number of disease states. Proteomic profiling of urinary exosomes has revealed a number of proteins known to be associated with specific renal diseases or blood pressure regulation [109]. To date, at least two exosomal associated proteins have been investigated as potential biomarkers in AKI, Na+/H+ exchanger isoform 3 (NHE3) and Fetuin-A [110, 111]. NHE3 has been identified as the most abundant sodium transporter in the renal tubule, responsible for the proximal reabsorption of 60 – 70% of filtered sodium and bicarbonate in mice [110, 112]. NHE3 is localized to the apical membrane and intracellular vesicular compartment of renal proximal tubular cells as well as the apical membrane of the thick and thin ascending limb cells [113-115]. McKee et al. demonstrated that NHE3 as well as two other sodium transporter proteins (bumetanide-sensitive Na-K-2Cl cotransporter [NKCC2] and thiazide sensitive Na-Cl cotransporter [NCC]) were readily detected in the urine of healthy rats in immunoblotting experiments [116]. Later studies confirmed the presence of NHE3 in urinary exosomes [117]. Given the well established increase in fractional excretion of sodium in the setting of tubular injury, du Cheyron et al. hypothesized that urinary NHE3 excretion may serve as a specific marker of AKI [110]. In their study of 68 critically ill adults, they performed semi-quantitative immunoblotting on urine membrane fractions and found urinary NHE-3 excretion to be a useful marker in discriminating between control patients, those with prerenal azotemia, those with acute glomerular disease, and those with ischemic/nephrotoxic ATN [110]. It was recently reported, however, that specimen storage and processing in this study were suboptimal, possibly resulting in increased degradation and decreased recovery of NHE3 prior to protein quantification [117]. Fetuin-A is an acute phase protein synthesized in the liver and secreted into the circulation, where it has been implicated in several diverse functions, including bone resorption, regulation of insulin activity and hepatocyte growth factor activity, response to inflammation and inhibition of ectopic mineralization [118]. Zhou et al. identified urinary exosomal fetuin-A (EF-A) to be markedly increased in rats following cisplatin injection. Urinary EF-A increased greater than 50-fold at day 2, preceding changes in serum creatinine and histologic evidence of tubule damage by 1 day, and remained elevated until day 5, when tubule damage was most severe [111]. Increased urinary EF-A was additionally noted following I/R injury, but not in the setting of prerenal azotemia [111]. In a limited number of clinical specimens (n = 9), urinary EF-A was found to be much higher in ICU patients with AKI compared to ICU patients without AKI and healthy volunteers [111]. Immunohistochemical staining localized fetuin-A to the cytoplasm of damaged proximal tubule cells with higher concentrations evident with increasing severity of injury [111]. Although the function of fetuin-A in AKI remains unknown, it may play a role in tubule cell apoptosis. Significant issues with assay throughput and sensitivity currently exist in the quantification of exosomal associated proteins, limiting their practical use in large scale studies of AKI. Published studies have exclusively employed immunoblotting, a labor intensive and semi-quantitative method. In addition, isolation of urinary exosomes requires ultracentrifugation of specimens, a process that takes 1 − 2 hours and several steps [109-111, 116, 117]. Fortunately, Cheruvanky et al. [119] recently reported that exosomal isolation may be simplified considerably through the use of a commercially available nanomembrane concentrator.

Other Biomarkers

A number of other biomarkers of AKI have been proposed, but require further characterization to determine clinical utility. Cysteine-rich protein (Cyr61) was found to be rapidly induced and excreted into the lumen of the proximal tubules following bilateral I/R injury in rats; however, levels fell quickly despite progression of injury [120]. Clusterin is a multifaceted glycoprotein that has been studied extensively in a variety of preclinical AKI models, including I/R injury, nephrotoxicant induced injury, and unilateral ureteral obstruction [121-125]. There are currently no clinical studies evaluating urinary clusterin as a potential biomarker in AKI. Osteopontin, a potent chemoattractant of mononuclear cells, has been investigated extensively in animals and humans. Immunohistochemical and in situ-hybridization studies have demonstrated upregulated expression in a number of conditions associated with AKI, including I/R injury, nephrotoxicant exposure, and renal allograft rejection [126-131]. There are currently no published studies evaluating urinary osteopontin as a potential biomarker in AKI, although it is known to be excreted in the urine and there are commercially available ELISA kits that may be used for quantification.

Future Directions

Efforts to identify biomarkers to assist with the early diagnosis of AKI have yielded many promising candidates. To date, most studies have emphasized discovery, characterization, and validation of individual biomarkers using a single model of kidney injury. This approach is necessary in the initial stages of biomarker development; however, translation to general clinical applicability requires considerable additional work. In the clinical setting, an ideal biomarker for the detection AKI is one that is easily obtained, easily and rapidly measured, sensitive to minor disturbances in normal function, site specific, highly correlated with the degree of injury, and indicative of injury progression and regression. A single biomarker is rarely adequate to clearly define a particular pathologic state [132, 133]. Given inherent renal heterogeneity and the disparate settings under which kidney injury occurs, a panel of carefully selected biomarkers may prove to be most appropriate. Development of such a panel will require large, well designed prospective studies comparing multiple biomarkers in the same set of urine samples over extended time courses. Such studies will allow temporal patterns of biomarker elevation to be established, patterns that may be specific to the mechanism of injury (nephrotoxicant, ischemia, allograft rejection, etc.), population of interest (elderly, pediatric, etc.), and/or co-occurring disease states (diabetes, heart disease, sepsis, etc.).

As biomarker panels emerge for the detection of AKI, considerable effort will need to be directed toward developing technologies that will permit the rapid detection and quantification necessary in clinical practice. Presently, most candidate biomarkers are measured by ELISA, a technique that is not only time and labor intensive but also does not allow multiple biomarkers to be assessed simultaneously in the same sample. Our group has developed assays for KIM-1 and NGAL quantification using a microbead platform, a particle based flow cytometric assay with multiplexing capabilities [33]; however, it still requires several hours to perform. Recent developments in nanotechnology may eventually allow for bedside detection. Zheng et al. [134] used a multiplexed electrical detection nanowire sensor array to detect multiple markers for prostate cancer in serum. Similar technology may eventually allow for continuous online monitoring for patients at risk for AKI in the ICU setting.

Conclusion

AKI is a common condition associated with considerable morbidity and mortality. Despite impressive advances in our understanding of the pathophysiology of AKI and optimization of care for those with AKI, outcomes have remained little changed over the last 50 years.

Urinary biomarkers have been identified that are highly sensitive and specific for kidney injury. These biomarkers will enable earlier diagnosis of kidney injury, will enable prognosis of outcome, and will provide strategies for stratification of patients for interventional trials. Further characterization and validation of individual biomarkers and biomarker panels in AKI will identify the most useful biomarkers ultimately resulting in improved patient outcomes (Figure 2).

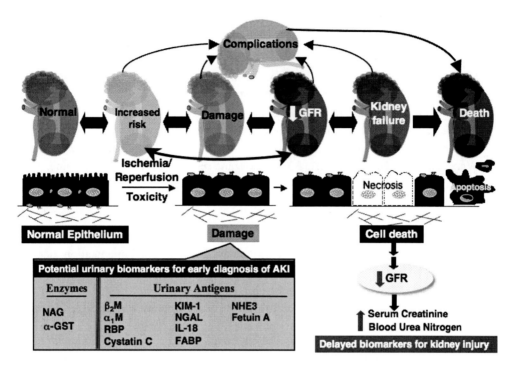

Figure 2. Acute kidney injury exists along a continuum with severity of injury closely correlated with associated complications and eventual outcome. AKI can be conceptualized as a number of reversible stages, initiating with increased risk and damage and progressing to decreased glomerular filtration rate (GFR) to eventual kidney failure and death. It should also be noted that diminished renal perfusion may result in decreased GFR in the absence of intrinsic damage (prerenal azotemia). Traditionally used markers of renal injury, such as blood urea nitrogen (BUN) and creatinine (CR), are insensitive, nonspecific and do not adequately differentiate between the different stages of AKI resulting in delayed diagnosis and intervention. Urinary biomarkers of AKI will facilitate earlier diagnosis and differentiated preventative and therapeutic strategies, ultimately resulting in fewer complications and improved outcomes. (Adapted from Vaidya, Ferguson, and Bonventre, Annual Reviews of Pharmacology and Toxicology, 2007; Mehta, R.L., Kellum, J.A., Shah, S., Molitoris, B.A., Ronco, C., Warnock, D., and Levin, A. 2006. AKIN: Acute Kidney Injury Network: report of an initiative. In *AKIN Summit*. Amsterdam.).

References

[1]   Bonventre, J.V., and Weinberg, J.M. 2003. Recent advances in the pathophysiology of ischemic acute renal failure. *J. Am. Soc. Nephrol.* 14:2199-2210.

[2]   Schrier, R.W., Wang, W., Poole, B., and Mitra, A. 2004. Acute renal failure: definitions, diagnosis, pathogenesis, and therapy. *J. Clin. Invest.* 114:5-14.

[3]   Bonventre, J.V. 2003. Dedifferentiation and proliferation of surviving epithelial cells in acute renal failure. *J. Am. Soc. Nephrol.* 14 Suppl 1:S55-61.

[4]   Thadhani, R., Pascual, M., and Bonventre, J.V. 1996. Acute renal failure. *N. Engl. J. Med.* 334:1448-1460.

[5]   Liu, K.D., Matthay, M.A., and Chertow, G.M. 2006. Evolving practices in critical care and potential implications for management of acute kidney injury. *Clin. J. Am. Soc. Nephrol.* 1:869-873.

[6]   Martin, G.S., Mannino, D.M., Eaton, S., and Moss, M. 2003. The epidemiology of sepsis in the United States from 1979 through 2000. *N. Engl. J. Med.* 348:1546-1554.

[7]   2000. Ventilation with lower tidal volumes as compared with traditional tidal volumes for acute lung injury and the acute respiratory distress syndrome. The Acute Respiratory Distress Syndrome Network. *N. Engl. J. Med.* 342:1301-1308.

[8]   Ware, L.B., and Matthay, M.A. 2000. The acute respiratory distress syndrome. *N. Engl. J. Med.* 342:1334-1349.

[9]   Mehta, R.L., and Chertow, G.M. 2003. Acute renal failure definitions and classification: time for change? *J. Am. Soc. Nephrol.* 14:2178-2187.

[10] Chertow, G.M., Lee, J., Kuperman, G.J., Burdick, E., Horsky, J., Seger, D.L., Lee, R., Mekala, A., Song, J., Komaroff, A.L., et al. 2001. Guided medication dosing for inpatients with renal insufficiency. *Jama* 286:2839-2844.

[11] Edwards, N., Honemann, D., Burley, D., and Navarro, M. 1994. Refinement of the Medicare diagnosis-related groups to incorporate a measure of severity. *Health Care Financ Rev* 16:45-64.

[12] Hou, S.H., Bushinsky, D.A., Wish, J.B., Cohen, J.J., and Harrington, J.T. 1983. Hospital-acquired renal insufficiency: a prospective study. *Am. J. Med.* 74:243-248.

[13] Nash, K., Hafeez, A., and Hou, S. 2002. Hospital-acquired renal insufficiency. *Am. J. Kidney Dis.* 39:930-936.

[14] Shusterman, N., Strom, B.L., Murray, T.G., Morrison, G., West, S.L., and Maislin, G. 1987. Risk factors and outcome of hospital-acquired acute renal failure. Clinical epidemiologic study. *Am. J. Med.* 83:65-71.

[15] Liangos, O., Wald, R., O'Bell, J.W., Price, L., Pereira, B.J., and Jaber, B.L. 2006. Epidemiology and outcomes of acute renal failure in hospitalized patients: a national survery. *Clin. J. Am. Soc. Nephrol.* 1:43-51.

[16] Chertow, G.M., Levy, E.M., Hammermeister, K.E., Grover, F., and Daley, J. 1998. Independent association between acute renal failure and mortality following cardiac surgery. *Am. J. Med.* 104:343-348.

[17] de Mendonca, A., Vincent, J.L., Suter, P.M., Moreno, R., Dearden, N.M., Antonelli, M., Takala, J., Sprung, C., and Cantraine, F. 2000. Acute renal failure in the ICU: risk factors and outcome evaluated by the SOFA score. *Intensive Care Med.* 26:915-921.

[18] Ympa, Y.P., Sakr, Y., Reinhart, K., and Vincent, J.L. 2005. Has mortality from acute renal failure decreased? A systematic review of the literature. *Am. J. Med.* 118:827-832.

[19] Uchino, S., Kellum, J.A., Bellomo, R., Doig, G.S., Morimatsu, H., Morgera, S., Schetz, M., Tan, I., Bouman, C., Macedo, E., et al. 2005. Acute renal failure in critically ill patients: a multinational, multicenter study. *Jama* 294:813-818.

[20] Hui-Stickle, S., Brewer, E.D., and Goldstein, S.L. 2005. Pediatric ARF epidemiology at a tertiary care center from 1999 to 2001. *Am. J. Kidney Dis.* 45:96-101.

[21] Counahan, R., Cameron, J.S., Ogg, C.S., Spurgeon, P., Williams, D.G., Winder, E., and Chantler, C. 1977. Presentation, management, complications, and outcome of acute renal failure in childhood: five years' experience. *Br. Med. J.* 1:599-602.

[22] Askenazi, D.J., Feig, D.I., Graham, N.M., Hui-Stickle, S., and Goldstein, S.L. 2006. 3-5 year longitudinal follow-up of pediatric patients after acute renal failure. *Kidney Int.* 69:184-189.

[23] Ronco, C., Kellum, J.A., and Mehta, R. 2001. Acute dialysis quality initiative (ADQI). *Nephrol. Dial Transplant* 16:1555-1558.

[24] Kellum, J.A., Levin, N., Bouman, C., and Lameire, N. 2002. Developing a consensus classification system for acute renal failure. *Curr. Opin. Crit. Care* 8:509-514.

[25] Bellomo, R., Ronco, C., Kellum, J.A., Mehta, R.L., and Palevsky, P. 2004. Acute renal failure - definition, outcome measures, animal models, fluid therapy and information technology needs: the Second International Consensus Conference of the Acute Dialysis Quality Initiative (ADQI) Group. *Crit Care* 8:R204-212.

[26] Warnock, D.G. 2005. Towards a definition and classification of acute kidney injury. *J. Am. Soc. Nephrol.* 16:3149-3150.

[27] Chertow, G.M., Burdick, E., Honour, M., Bonventre, J.V., and Bates, D.W. 2005. Acute kidney injury, mortality, length of stay, and costs in hospitalized patients. *J. Am. Soc. Nephrol.* 16:3365-3370.

[28] Lassnigg, A., Schmidlin, D., Mouhieddine, M., Bachmann, L.M., Druml, W., Bauer, P., and Hiesmayr, M. 2004. Minimal changes of serum creatinine predict prognosis in patients after cardiothoracic surgery: a prospective cohort study. *J. Am. Soc. Nephrol.* 15:1597-1605.

[29] Mehta, R.L., Kellum, J.A., Shah, S., Molitoris, B.A., Ronco, C., Warnock, D., and Levin, A. 2006. AKIN: Acute Kidney Injury Network: report of an initiative. In *AKIN Summit*. Amsterdam.

[30] Akcan-Arikan, A., Zapitelli, M., Loftus, L.,Washburn, K., Jefferson, S., Goldstein, S. 2007. Modified RIFLE criteria in critically ill children with acute kidney injury. *Kidney Int.* 71:1028-1035..

[31] Star, R.A. 1998. Treatment of acute renal failure. *Kidney Int.* 54:1817-1831.

[32] Moran, S.M., and Myers, B.D. 1985. Course of acute renal failure studied by a model of creatinine kinetics. *Kidney Int.* 27:928-937.

[33] Vaidya, V.S. and Bonventre, J.V. 2006. Mechanistic biomarkers for cytotoxic acute kidney injury. *Expert. Opin. Drug Metab. Toxicol.* 2:697-713.

[34] Trof, R.J., Di Maggio, F., Leemreis, J., and Groeneveld, A.B. 2006. Biomarkers of acute renal injury and renal failure. *Shock* 26:245-253.

[35] Emeigh Hart, S.G. 2005. Assessment of renal injury in vivo. *J. Pharmacol. Toxicol. Methods* 52:30-45.

[36] Goldstein, S.L. 2006. Pediatric acute kidney injury: it's time for real progress. *Pediatr. Nephrol.* 21:891-895.

[37] D'Amico, G., and Bazzi, C. 2003. Urinary protein and enzyme excretion as markers of tubular damage. *Curr. Opin. Nephrol. Hypertens* 12:639-643.

[38] Westhuyzen, J., Endre, Z.H., Reece, G., Reith, D.M., Saltissi, D., and Morgan, T.J. 2003. Measurement of tubular enzymuria facilitates early detection of acute renal impairment in the intensive care unit. *Nephrol. Dial. Transplant.* 18:543-551.

[39] Mukhopadhyay, B., Chinchole, S., Lobo, V., Gang, S., and Rajapurkar, M. 2004. Enzymuria pattern in early port renal tranplant period: diagnostic usefulness in graft dysfunction. *Indian Journal of Clinical Biochemistry* 19:14-19.

[40] Bazzi, C., Petrini, C., Rizza, V., Arrigo, G., Napodano, P., Paparella, M., and D'Amico, G. 2002. Urinary N-acetyl-beta-glucosaminidase excretion is a marker of tubular cell dysfunction and a predictor of outcome in primary glomerulonephritis. *Nephrol. Dial. Transplant.* 17:1890-1896.

[41] Ikenaga, H., Suzuki, H., Ishii, N., Itoh, H., and Saruta, T. 1993. Enzymuria in non-insulin-dependent diabetic patients: signs of tubular cell dysfunction. *Clin. Sci. (Lond)* 84:469-475.

[42] Ascione, R., Lloyd, C.T., Underwood, M.J., Gomes, W.J., and Angelini, G.D. 1999. On-pump versus off-pump coronary revascularization: evaluation of renal function. *Ann. Thorac. Surg.* 68:493-498.

[43] Chew, S.L., Lins, R.L., Daelemans, R., Nuyts, G.D., and De Broe, M.E. 1993. Urinary enzymes in acute renal failure. *Nephrol. Dial. Transplant.* 8:507-511.

[44] Liangos, O., Perianayagam, M.C., Vaidya, V.S., Han, W.K., Wald, R., Tighiouart, H., MacKinnon, R.W., Li, L., Balakrishnan, V.S., Pereira, B.J., et al. 2007. Urinary N-acetyl-beta-(D)-glucosaminidase activity and kidney injury molecule-1 level are associated with adverse outcomes in acute renal failure. *J. Am. Soc. Nephrol.* 18:904-912.

[45] Bondiou, M.T., Bourbouze, R., Bernard, M., Percheron, F., Perez-Gonzalez, N., and Cabezas, J.A. 1985. Inhibition of A and B N-acetyl-beta-D-glucosaminidase urinary isoenzymes by urea. *Clin. Chim. Acta* 149:67-73.

[46] Usuda, K., Kono, K., Dote, T., Nishiura, K., Miyata, K., Nishiura, H., Shimahara, M., and Sugimoto, K. 1998. Urinary biomarkers monitoring for experimental fluoride nephrotoxicity. *Arch. Toxicol.* 72:104-109.

[47] D'Amico, G., and Bazzi, C. 2003. Pathophysiology of proteinuria. *Kidney Int.* 63:809-825.

[48] Tolkoff-Rubin, N.E., Rubin, R.H., and Bonventre, J.V. 1988. Noninvasive renal diagnostic studies. *Clin. Lab. Med.* 8:507-526.

[49] Miyata, T., Jadoul, M., Kurokawa, K., and Van Ypersele de Strihou, C. 1998. Beta-2 microglobulin in renal disease. *J. Am. Soc. Nephrol.* 9:1723-1735.

[50] Chapelsky, M.C., Nix, D.E., Cavanaugh, J.C., Wilton, J.H., Norman, A., and Schentag, J.J. 1992. Renal tubular enzyme effects of clarithromycin in comparison with gentamicin and placebo in volunteers. *Drug Saf.* 7:304-309.

[51] Dehne, M.G., Boldt, J., Heise, D., Sablotzki, A., and Hempelmann, G. 1995. [Tamm-Horsfall protein, alpha-1- and beta-2-microglobulin as kidney function markers in heart surgery]. *Anaesthesist* 44:545-551.

[52] Fernandez, F., de Miguel, M.D., Barrio, V., and Mallol, J. 1988. Beta-2-microglobulin as an index of renal function after cardiopulmonary bypass surgery in children. *Child Nephrol. Urol.* 9:326-330.

[53] Schaub, S., Wilkins, J.A., Antonovici, M., Krokhin, O., Weiler, T., Rush, D., and Nickerson, P. 2005. Proteomic-based identification of cleaved urinary beta2-microglobulin as a potential marker for acute tubular injury in renal allografts. *Am. J. Transplant.* 5:729-738.

[54] Herget-Rosenthal, S., Poppen, D., Husing, J., Marggraf, G., Pietruck, F., Jakob, H.G., Philipp, T., and Kribben, A. 2004. Prognostic value of tubular proteinuria and enzymuria in nonoliguric acute tubular necrosis. *Clin. Chem.* 50:552-558.

[55] Yu, H., Yanagisawa, Y., Forbes, M.A., Cooper, E.H., Crockson, R.A., and MacLennan, I.C. 1983. Alpha-1-microglobulin: an indicator protein for renal tubular function. *J. Clin. Pathol.* 36:253-259.

[56] Wolf, M.W., and Boldt, J. 2007. Kidney specific proteins: markers for detection of renal dysfunction after cardiac surgery? *Clin. Res. Cardiol. Suppl.* 2:S103-S107.

[57] Ojala, R., Ala-Houhala, M., Harmoinen, A.P., Luukkaala, T., Uotila, J., and Tammela, O. 2006. Tubular proteinuria in pre-term and full-term infants. *Pediatr. Nephrol.* 21:68-73.

[58] Bernard, A.M., Vyskocil, A.A., Mahieu, P., and Lauwerys, R.R. 1987. Assessment of urinary retinol-binding protein as an index of proximal tubular injury. *Clin. Chem.* 33:775-779.

[59] Roberts, D.S., Haycock, G.B., Dalton, R.N., Turner, C., Tomlinson, P., Stimmler, L., and Scopes, J.W. 1990. Prediction of acute renal failure after birth asphyxia. *Arch. Dis. Child* 65:1021-1028.

[60] Shlipak, M.G., Sarnak, M.J., Katz, R., Fried, L.F., Seliger, S.L., Newman, A.B., Siscovick, D.S., and Stehman-Breen, C. 2005. Cystatin C and the risk of death and cardiovascular events among elderly persons. *N. Engl. J. Med.* 352:2049-2060.

[61] Conti, M., Moutereau, S., Zater, M., Lallali, K., Durrbach, A., Manivet, P., Eschwege, P., and Loric, S. 2006. Urinary cystatin C as a specific marker of tubular dysfunction. *Clin. Chem. Lab. Med.* 44:288-291.

[62] Uchida, K., and Gotoh, A. 2002. Measurement of cystatin-C and creatinine in urine. *Clin. Chim. Acta* 323:121-128.

[63] Muller, F., Bernard, M.A., Benkirane, A., Ngo, S., Lortat-Jacob, S., Oury, J.F., and Dommergues, M. 1999. Fetal urine cystatin C as a predictor of postnatal renal function in bilateral uropathies. *Clin. Chem.* 45:2292-2293.

[64] Ichimura, T., Bonventre, J.V., Bailly, V., Wei, H., Hession, C.A., Cate, R.L., and Sanicola, M. 1998. Kidney injury molecule-1 (KIM-1), a putative epithelial cell adhesion molecule containing a novel immunoglobulin domain, is up-regulated in renal cells after injury. *J. Biol. Chem.* 273:4135-4142.

[65] Amin, R.P., Vickers, A.E., Sistare, F., Thompson, K.L., Roman, R.J., Lawton, M., Kramer, J., Hamadeh, H.K., Collins, J., Grissom, S., et al. 2004. Identification of putative gene based markers of renal toxicity. *Environ. Health Perspect.* 112:465-479.

[66] Bailly, V., Zhang, Z., Meier, W., Cate, R., Sanicola, M., and Bonventre, J.V. 2002. Shedding of kidney injury molecule-1, a putative adhesion protein involved in renal regeneration. *J. Biol. Chem.* 277:39739-39748.

[67] Goering, P.L., Vaidya, V.S., Brown, R.P., Vakili, Z., Rosenzweig, B.A., Johnson, A.M., Thompson, K.L., and Bonventre, J.V. 2006. Kidney injury molecule-1 (kim-1) expression in Kidney and urine following acute exposure To gentamicin and mercury. *The Toxicologist* 90:341.

[68] Humphreys, B.D., Vaidya, V.S., Samarakoon, R., Hentschel, D.M., Park, K.M., and Bonventre, J.V. 2005. Early and sustained expression of Kidney injury molecule-1 (Kim-1) after unilateral ureteral obstruction. *J. Am. Soc. Nephrol.* 16:425A.

[69] Ichimura, T., Hung, C.C., Yang, S.A., Stevens, J.L., and Bonventre, J.V. 2004. Kidney injury molecule-1: a tissue and urinary biomarker for nephrotoxicant-induced renal injury. *Am. J. Physiol. Renal Physiol.* 286:F552-563.

[70] Prozialeck, W.C., Vaidya, V.S., Johnson, A.M., Liu, J., Waalkes, M.P., Edwards, J.R., Diamantakos, E., Lamar, P.C., Theusch, J., and Bonventre, J.V. 2006. Kidney injury molecule-1 (kim-1) as an early biomarker of cadmium (cd) nephrotoxicity. *The Toxicologist* 90:340.

[71] Vaidya, V.S., Ramirez, V., Bobadilla, N.A., and Bonventre, J.V. 2005. A microfluidics based assay to measure Kidney Injury Molecule-1 (Kim-1) in the urine as a biomarker for early diagnosis of acute kidney injury. *J. Am. Soc. Nephrol.* 16:192A.

[72] Vaidya, V.S., Ramirez, V., Ichimura, T., Bobadilla, N.A., and Bonventre, J.V. 2006. Urinary kidney injury molecule-1: a sensitive quantitative biomarker for early detection of kidney tubular injury. *Am. J. Physiol. Renal Physiol.* 290:F517-529.

[73] Han, W.K., Bailly, V., Abichandani, R., Thadhani, R., and Bonventre, J.V. 2002. Kidney Injury Molecule-1 (KIM-1): a novel biomarker for human renal proximal tubule injury. *Kidney Int.* 62:237-244.

[73a] Liangos, O., Perianayagam, M.C., Vaidya, V.S., Han, W.K., Wald, R., Tighiouart, H., MacKinnon, R.W., Li, L., Balakrishnan, V.S., Pereira, B.J.G., Bonventre, J.V., Jaber, B.L. 2007. Urinary N-acetyl-B-glucosaminidase activity and and Kidney Injury Molecule-1 level are asssociated with adverse outcomes in acute renal failure. *J. Am. Soc. Nephrol.* 18:904-912.

[73b] van Timmeren, M.M., Vaidya, V.S., van Ree, R.M., Oterdoom, L.H., de Vries, A.P.J., Gans, R.O.B., van Goor, H., Stegemanm C.A., Bonventre, J.V., Bakker, S.J.L. 2007. High urinary excretion of Kidney Injury Molecule-1 is an independent predictor of graft loss in renal transplant recipients. *Transplantation* 84:1625-1630

[73c] Zhang, P.L., Rothblum, L.I., Han, W.K., Blasick, T.M., Potdar, S., Bonventre, J.V. 2008. Kidney Injury Molecule-1 in transplant biopsies is a sensitive measure of cell injury. *Kidney Int.* 73: 608-614.

[74] Borregaard, N., Sehested, M., Nielsen, B.S., Sengelov, H., and Kjeldsen, L. 1995. Biosynthesis of granule proteins in normal human bone marrow cells. Gelatinase is a marker of terminal neutrophil differentiation. *Blood* 85:812-817.

[75] Nielsen, B.S., Borregaard, N., Bundgaard, J.R., Timshel, S., Sehested, M., and Kjeldsen, L. 1996. Induction of NGAL synthesis in epithelial cells of human colorectal neoplasia and inflammatory bowel diseases. *Gut* 38:414-420.

[76] Cowland, J.B., and Borregaard, N. 1997. Molecular characterization and pattern of tissue expression of the gene for neutrophil gelatinase-associated lipocalin from humans. *Genomics* 45:17-23.

[77] Mishra, J., Ma, Q., Prada, A., Mitsnefes, M., Zahedi, K., Yang, J., Barasch, J., and Devarajan, P. 2003. Identification of neutrophil gelatinase-associated lipocalin as a novel early urinary biomarker for ischemic renal injury. *J. Am. Soc. Nephrol.* 14:2534-2543.

[78] Yang, J., Goetz, D., Li, J.Y., Wang, W., Mori, K., Setlik, D., Du, T., Erdjument-Bromage, H., Tempst, P., Strong, R., et al. 2002. An iron delivery pathway mediated by a lipocalin. *Mol. Cell* 10:1045-1056.

[78a] Schmidt-Ott, K.M., Mori, K., Kalandadze, A., Li, J.Y., Paragas, N., Nicholas, T., Devarajan, P., Barasch, J. 2006. Neutrophil gelatinase-associated lipocalin iron traffic in kidney epithelia. *Curr. Opin. Nephrol. Hypertens.* 15:442-449.

[78b] Schmidt-Ott, K.M., Mori, K., Li, J.Y., Kalandadze, A., Cohen, D.J., Devarajan, P., Barasch, J. 2006. Dual action of neutrophil-gelatinase-associated lipocalin. *J. Am. Soc. Nephrol.* 18:407-413.

[79] Mishra, J., Mori, K., Ma, Q., Kelly, C., Barasch, J., and Devarajan, P. 2004. Neutrophil gelatinase-associated lipocalin: a novel early urinary biomarker for cisplatin nephrotoxicity. *Am. J. Nephrol.* 24:307-315.

[80] Mishra, J., Dent, C., Tarabishi, R., Mitsnefes, M.M., Ma, Q., Kelly, C., Ruff, S.M., Zahedi, K., Shao, M., Bean, J., et al. 2005. Neutrophil gelatinase-associated lipocalin (NGAL) as a biomarker for acute renal injury after cardiac surgery. *Lancet* 365:1231-1238.

[81] Wagener, G., Jan, M., Kim, M., Mori, K., Barasch, J.M., Sladen, R.N., and Lee, H.T. 2006. Association between increases in urinary neutrophil gelatinase-associated lipocalin and acute renal dysfunction after adult cardiac surgery. *Anesthesiology* 105:485-491.

[82] Trachtman, H., Christen, E., Cnaan, A., Patrick, J., Mai, V., Mishra, J., Jain, A., Bullington, N., and Devarajan, P. 2006. Urinary neutrophil gelatinase-associated lipocalcin in D+HUS: a novel marker of renal injury. *Pediatr. Nephrol.* 21:989-994.

[83] Ohlsson, S., Wieslander, J., and Segelmark, M. 2003. Increased circulating levels of proteinase 3 in patients with anti-neutrophilic cytoplasmic autoantibodies-associated systemic vasculitis in remission. *Clin. Exp. Immunol.* 131:528-535.

[84] Xu, S.Y., Pauksen, K., and Venge, P. 1995. Serum measurements of human neutrophil lipocalin (HNL) discriminate between acute bacterial and viral infections. *Scand. J. Clin. Lab. Invest.* 55:125-131.

[84a] Carlson, M., Raab, Y., Seveus, L., Xu, S., Hallgren, R., Venge, P. 2002. Human neutrophil lipocalin is a unique marker of inflammation in ulcerative colitis and proctitis. *Gut* 50:501-506.

[84b] Jonsson, P., Stahl, M.L., Ohlsson, K. 1999. Extracorporeal circulation causes relaease of neturophil gelatinase-associated lipocalin. *Mediators Inflamm.* 8:169-171.

[85] Ghayur, T., Banerjee, S., Hugunin, M., Butler, D., Herzog, L., Carter, A., Quintal, L., Sekut, L., Talanian, R., Paskind, M., et al. 1997. Caspase-1 processes IFN-gamma-inducing factor and regulates LPS-induced IFN-gamma production. *Nature* 386:619-623.

[86] Gracie, J.A., Robertson, S.E., and McInnes, I.B. 2003. Interleukin-18. *J. Leukoc. Biol.* 73:213-224.

[87] Gu, Y., Kuida, K., Tsutsui, H., Ku, G., Hsiao, K., Fleming, M.A., Hayashi, N., Higashino, K., Okamura, H., Nakanishi, K., et al. 1997. Activation of interferon-gamma inducing factor mediated by interleukin-1beta converting enzyme. *Science* 275:206-209.

[88] Pomerantz, B.J., Reznikov, L.L., Harken, A.H., and Dinarello, C.A. 2001. Inhibition of caspase 1 reduces human myocardial ischemic dysfunction via inhibition of IL-18 and IL-1beta. *Proc. Natl. Acad. Sci. USA* 98:2871-2876.

[89] Melnikov, V.Y., Ecder, T., Fantuzzi, G., Siegmund, B., Lucia, M.S., Dinarello, C.A., Schrier, R.W., and Edelstein, C.L. 2001. Impaired IL-18 processing protects caspase-1-deficient mice from ischemic acute renal failure. *J. Clin. Invest* 107:1145-1152.

[90] Melnikov, V.Y., Faubel, S., Siegmund, B., Lucia, M.S., Ljubanovic, D., and Edelstein, C.L. 2002. Neutrophil-independent mechanisms of caspase-1- and IL-18-mediated ischemic acute tubular necrosis in mice. *J. Clin. Invest* 110:1083-1091.

[91] Parikh, C.R., Jani, A., Melnikov, V.Y., Faubel, S., and Edelstein, C.L. 2004. Urinary interleukin-18 is a marker of human acute tubular necrosis. *Am. J. Kidney Dis.* 43:405-414.

[92] Striz, I., Krasna, E., Honsova, E., Lacha, J., Petrickova, K., Jaresova, M., Lodererova, A., Bohmova, R., Valhova, S., Slavcev, A., et al. 2005. Interleukin 18 (IL-18) upregulation in acute rejection of kidney allograft. *Immunol. Lett.* 99:30-35.

[93] Parikh, C.R., Abraham, E., Ancukiewicz, M., and Edelstein, C.L. 2005. Urine IL-18 is an early diagnostic marker for acute kidney injury and predicts mortality in the intensive care unit. *J. Am. Soc. Nephrol* .16:3046-3052.

[94] Pelsers, M.M., Hermens, W.T., and Glatz, J.F. 2005. Fatty acid-binding proteins as plasma markers of tissue injury. *Clin. Chim. Acta* 352:15-35.

[95] Oyama, Y., Takeda, T., Hama, H., Tanuma, A., Iino, N., Sato, K., Kaseda, R., Ma, M., Yamamoto, T., Fujii, H., et al. 2005. Evidence for megalin-mediated proximal tubular uptake of L-FABP, a carrier of potentially nephrotoxic molecules. *Lab. Invest* 85:522-531.

[96] Ek-Von Mentzer, B.A., Zhang, F., and Hamilton, J.A. 2001. Binding of 13-HODE and 15-HETE to phospholipid bilayers, albumin, and intracellular fatty acid binding proteins. implications for transmembrane and intracellular transport and for protection from lipid peroxidation. *J. Biol. Chem.* 276:15575-15580.

[97] Maatman, R.G., van de Westerlo, E.M., van Kuppevelt, T.H., and Veerkamp, J.H. 1992. Molecular identification of the liver- and the heart-type fatty acid-binding proteins in human and rat kidney. Use of the reverse transcriptase polymerase chain reaction. *Biochem J.* 288 (Pt 1):285-290.

[98] Maatman, R.G., Van Kuppevelt, T.H., and Veerkamp, J.H. 1991. Two types of fatty acid-binding protein in human kidney. Isolation, characterization and localization. *Biochem J.* 273 (Pt 3):759-766.

[99] Gok, M.A., Pelsers, M., Glatz, J.F., Shenton, B.K., Peaston, R., Cornell, C., and Talbot, D. 2003. Use of two biomarkers of renal ischemia to assess machine-perfused non-heart-beating donor kidneys. *Clin. Chem.* 49:172-175.

[100] Gok, M.A., Pelzers, M., Glatz, J.F., Shenton, B.K., Buckley, P.E., Peaston, R., Cornell, C., Mantle, D., Soomro, N., Jaques, B.C., et al. 2003. Do tissue damage biomarkers used to assess machine-perfused NHBD kidneys predict long-term renal function post-transplant? *Clin. Chim. Acta* 338:33-43.

[101] Kamijo, A., Sugaya, T., Hikawa, A., Okada, M., Okumura, F., Yamanouchi, M., Honda, A., Okabe, M., Fujino, T., Hirata, Y., et al. 2004. Urinary excretion of fatty acid-binding protein reflects stress overload on the proximal tubules. *Am. J. Pathol.* 165:1243-1255.

[102] Kamijo, A., Sugaya, T., Hikawa, A., Yamanouchi, M., Hirata, Y., Ishimitsu, T., Numabe, A., Takagi, M., Hayakawa, H., Tabei, F., et al. 2006. Urinary liver-type fatty acid binding protein as a useful biomarker in chronic kidney disease. *Mol Cell Biochem* 284:175-182.

[103] Suzuki, K., Babazono, T., Murata, H., and Iwamoto, Y. 2005. Clinical significance of urinary liver-type fatty acid-binding protein in patients with diabetic nephropathy. *Diabetes Care* 28:2038-2039.

[104] Nakamura, T., Sugaya, T., and Koide, H. 2007. Angiotensin II receptor antagonist reduces urinary liver-type fatty acid-binding protein levels in patients with diabetic nephropathy and chronic renal failure. *Diabetologia* 50:490-492.

[105] Nakamura, T., Sugaya, T., Ebihara, I., and Koide, H. 2005. Urinary liver-type fatty acid-binding protein: discrimination between IgA nephropathy and thin basement membrane nephropathy. *Am. J. Nephrol.* 25:447-450.

[106] Nakamura, T., Sugaya, T., Node, K., Ueda, Y., and Koide, H. 2006. Urinary excretion of liver-type fatty acid-binding protein in contrast medium-induced nephropathy. *Am. J. Kidney Dis.* 47:439-444.

[107] Yamamoto T., Noiri, E., Ono, Y., Doi, K., Negishi, K., Kamijo, A., Kimura, K., Fujita, T., Kinukawa, T., Taniguchi, H., Nakamura, K., Goto, M., Shinozaki, N., Ohshima, S., and Sugaya, T. 2007. Renal L-type Fatty Acid binding protein in acute ischemic injury. *J. Am. Soc. Nephrol.* 18:2894-2902.

[107a] Ferguson, M., Vaidya, V, Waikar, S., Collings, F., Sunderland, K., Gioules, C., Bonventre, J. Liver-type fatty acid-binding protein (L-FABP): a novel urinary biomarker of acute kidney injury. 2007. *J. Am. Soc. Nephrol.* 18:41A-42A.

[107b] Portilla D., Dent, C., Sugaya, T., Nagothu, K., Kundl, I., Moore, P., Noiri, E., Devarajan, P. 2008. Liver fatty acid-binding protein as a biomarker of acute kidney injury after cardiac surgery. *Kidney Int.* 73:465-472.

[108] Hoorn, E.J., Pisitkun, T., Zietse, R., Gross, P., Frokiaer, J., Wang, N.S., Gonzales, P.A., Star, R.A., and Knepper, M.A. 2005. Prospects for urinary proteomics: exosomes as a source of urinary biomarkers. *Nephrology (Carlton)* 10:283-290.

[109] Pisitkun, T., Shen, R.F., and Knepper, M.A. 2004. Identification and proteomic profiling of exosomes in human urine. *Proc. Natl. Acad. Sci. USA* 101:13368-13373.

[110] du Cheyron, D., Daubin, C., Poggioli, J., Ramakers, M., Houillier, P., Charbonneau, P., and Paillard, M. 2003. Urinary measurement of Na+/H+ exchanger isoform 3 (NHE3) protein as new marker of tubule injury in critically ill patients with ARF. *Am. J. Kidney Dis.* 42:497-506.

[111] Zhou, H., Pisitkun, T., Aponte, A., Yuen, P.S., Hoffert, J.D., Yasuda, H., Hu, X., Chawla, L., Shen, R.F., Knepper, M.A., et al. 2006. Exosomal Fetuin-A identified by proteomics: a novel urinary biomarker for detecting acute kidney injury. *Kidney Int.* 70:1847-1857.

[112] Wang, T., Yang, C.L., Abbiati, T., Schultheis, P.J., Shull, G.E., Giebisch, G., and Aronson, P.S. 1999. Mechanism of proximal tubule bicarbonate absorption in NHE3 null mice. *Am J Physiol* 277:F298-302.

[113] Attmane-Elakeb, A., Chambrey, R., Tsimaratos, M., Leviel, F., Blanchard, A., Warnock, D.G., Paillard, M., and Podevin, R.A. 1996. Isolation and characterization of luminal and basolateral plasma membrane vesicles from the medullary thick ascending loop of Henle. *Kidney Int.* 50:1051-1057.

[114] Biemesderfer, D., Rutherford, P.A., Nagy, T., Pizzonia, J.H., Abu-Alfa, A.K., and Aronson, P.S. 1997. Monoclonal antibodies for high-resolution localization of NHE3 in adult and neonatal rat kidney. *Am. J. Physiol.* 273:F289-299.

[115] Eladari, D., Leviel, F., Pezy, F., Paillard, M., and Chambrey, R. 2002. Rat proximal NHE3 adapts to chronic acid-base disorders but not to chronic changes in dietary NaCl intake. *Am. J. Physiol. Renal Physiol.* 282:F835-843.

[116] McKee, J.A., Kumar, S., Ecelbarger, C.A., Fernandez-Llama, P., Terris, J., and Knepper, M.A. 2000. Detection of Na(+) transporter proteins in urine. *J. Am. Soc. Nephrol.* 11:2128-2132.

[117] Zhou, H., Yuen, P.S., Pisitkun, T., Gonzales, P.A., Yasuda, H., Dear, J.W., Gross, P., Knepper, M.A., and Star, R.A. 2006. Collection, storage, preservation, and normalization of human urinary exosomes for biomarker discovery. *Kidney Int.* 69:1471-1476.

[118] Denecke, B., Graber, S., Schafer, C., Heiss, A., Woltje, M., and Jahnen-Dechent, W. 2003. Tissue distribution and activity testing suggest a similar but not identical function of fetuin-B and fetuin-A. *Biochem J.* 376:135-145.

[119] Cheruvanky, A., Zhou, H., Pisitkun, T., Kopp, J.B., Knepper, M.A., Yuen, P.S., and Star, R.A. 2007. Rapid isolation of urinary exosomal biomarkers using a nanomembrane ultrafiltration concentrator. *Am. J. Physiol. Renal Physiol.*

[120] Muramatsu, Y., Tsujie, M., Kohda, Y., Pham, B., Perantoni, A.O., Zhao, H., Jo, S.K., Yuen, P.S., Craig, L., Hu, X., et al. 2002. Early detection of cysteine rich protein 61 (CYR61, CCN1) in urine following renal ischemic reperfusion injury. *Kidney Int.* 62:1601-1610.

[121] Chevalier, R.L. 1996. Growth factors and apoptosis in neonatal ureteral obstruction. *J. Am. Soc. Nephrol.* 7:1098-1105.

[122] Kharasch, E.D., Schroeder, J.L., Bammler, T., Beyer, R., and Srinouanprachanh, S. 2006. Gene Expression Profiling of Nephrotoxicity from the Sevoflurane Degradation Product Fluoromethyl-2,2-difluoro-1-(trifluoromethyl)vinyl Ether ("Compound A") in Rats. *Toxicol Sci.* 90:419-431.

[123] Rosenberg, M.E., and Paller, M.S. 1991. Differential gene expression in the recovery from ischemic renal injury. *Kidney Int.* 39:1156-1161.

[124] Silkensen, J.R., Agarwal, A., Nath, K.A., Manivel, J.C., and Rosenberg, M.E. 1997. Temporal induction of clusterin in cisplatin nephrotoxicity. *J. Am. Soc. Nephrol.* 8:302-305.

[125] Witzgall, R., Brown, D., Schwarz, C., and Bonventre, J.V. 1994. Localization of proliferating cell nuclear antigen, vimentin, c-Fos, and clusterin in the postischemic kidney. Evidence for a heterogenous genetic response among nephron segments, and a large pool of mitotically active and dedifferentiated cells. *J. Clin. Invest.* 93:2175-2188.

[126] Alchi, B., Nishi, S., Kondo, D., Kaneko, Y., Matsuki, A., Imai, N., Ueno, M., Iguchi, S., Sakatsume, M., Narita, I., et al. 2005. Osteopontin expression in acute renal allograft rejection. *Kidney Int.* 67:886-896.

[127] Basile, D.P., Fredrich, K., Alausa, M., Vio, C.P., Liang, M., Rieder, M.R., Greene, A.S., and Cowley, A.W., Jr. 2005. Identification of persistently altered gene expression in the kidney after functional recovery from ischemic acute renal failure. *Am. J. Physiol. Renal Physiol.* 288:F953-963.

[128] Iguchi, S., Nishi, S., Ikegame, M., Hoshi, K., Yoshizawa, T., Kawashima, H., Arakawa, M., Ozawa, H., and Gejyo, F. 2004. Expression of osteopontin in cisplatin-induced tubular injury. *Nephron Exp Nephrol* 97:e96-105.

[129] Persy, V.P., Verstrepen, W.A., Ysebaert, D.K., De Greef, K.E., and De Broe, M.E. 1999. Differences in osteopontin up-regulation between proximal and distal tubules after renal ischemia/reperfusion. *Kidney Int* 56:601-611.

[130] Verstrepen, W.A., Persy, V.P., Verhulst, A., Dauwe, S., and De Broe, M.E. 2001. Renal osteopontin protein and mRNA upregulation during acute nephrotoxicity in the rat. *Nephrol. Dial. Transplant.* 16:712-724.

[131] Xie, Y., Nishi, S., Iguchi, S., Imai, N., Sakatsume, M., Saito, A., Ikegame, M., Iino, N., Shimada, H., Ueno, M., et al. 2001. Expression of osteopontin in gentamicin-induced acute tubular necrosis and its recovery process. *Kidney Int.* 59:959-974.

[132] Fliser, D., Novak, J., Thongboonkerd, V., Argiles, A., Jankowski, V., Girolami, M.A., Jankowski, J., and Mischak, H. 2007. Advances in Urinary Proteome Analysis and Biomarker Discovery. *J. Am. Soc. Nephrol.*

[133] Rifai, N., Gillette, M.A., and Carr, S.A. 2006. Protein biomarker discovery and validation: the long and uncertain path to clinical utility. *Nat. Biotechnol.* 24:971-983.

[134] Zheng, G., Patolsky, F., Cui, Y., Wang, W.U., and Lieber, C.M. 2005. Multiplexed electrical detection of cancer markers with nanowire sensor arrays. *Nat. Biotechnol.* 23:1294-1301.

[135] Holdt-Lehmann, B., Lehmann, A., Korten, G., Nagel, H., Nizze, H., and Schuff-Werner, P. 2000. Diagnostic value of urinary alanine aminopeptidase and N-acetyl-beta-D-glucosaminidase in comparison to alpha 1-microglobulin as a marker in evaluating tubular dysfunction in glomerulonephritis patients. *Clin. Chim. Acta* 297:93-102.

[136] Mueller, P.W., MacNeil, M.L., and Steinberg, K.K. 1986. Stabilization of alanine aminopeptidase, gamma glutamyltranspeptidase, and N-acetyl-beta-D-glucosaminidase activity in normal urines. *Arch. Environ. Contam. Toxicol.* 15:343-347.

[137] Rybak, M.J., Frankowski, J.J., Edwards, D.J., and Albrecht, L.M. 1987. Alanine aminopeptidase and beta 2-microglobulin excretion in patients receiving vancomycin and gentamicin. *Antimicrob Agents Chemother* 31:1461-1464.

[138] Jung, K., Pergande, M., Schroder, K., and Schreiber, G. 1982. Influence of pH on the activity of enzymes in urine at 37 degrees C. *Clin. Chem.* 28:1814.

[139] Nuyts, G.D., Yaqoob, M., Nouwen, E.J., Patrick, A.W., McClelland, P., MacFarlane, I.A., Bell, G.M., and De Broe, M.E. 1994. Human urinary intestinal alkaline phosphatase as an indicator of S3-segment-specific alterations in incipient diabetic nephropathy. *Nephrol. Dial. Transplant* 9:377-381.

[140] Cressey, G., Roberts, D.R., and Snowden, C.P. 2002. Renal tubular injury after infrarenal aortic aneurysm repair. *J. Cardiothorac. Vasc. Anesth.* 16:290-293.

[141] Eger, E.I., 2nd, Koblin, D.D., Bowland, T., Ionescu, P., Laster, M.J., Fang, Z., Gong, D., Sonner, J., and Weiskopf, R.B. 1997. Nephrotoxicity of sevoflurane versus desflurane anesthesia in volunteers. *Anesth. Analg.* 84:160-168.

[142] Van Kreel, B.K., Janssen, M.A., and Kootstra, G. 2002. Functional relationship of alpha-glutathione S-transferase and glutathione S-transferase activity in machine-preserved non-heart-beating donor kidneys. *Transpl. Int.* 15:546-549.

[143] Jung, K., and Grutzmann, K.D. 1988. Quality control material for activity determinations of urinary enzymes. *Clin. Biochem.* 21:53-57.

[144] Kamijo, A., Kimura, K., Sugaya, T., Yamanouchi, M., Hikawa, A., Hirano, N., Hirata, Y., Goto, A., and Omata, M. 2004. Urinary fatty acid-binding protein as a new clinical marker of the progression of chronic renal disease. *J. Lab. Clin. Med.* 143:23-30.

[145] Cowland, J.B., Sorensen, O.E., Sehested, M., and Borregaard, N. 2003. Neutrophil gelatinase-associated lipocalin is up-regulated in human epithelial cells by IL-1 beta, but not by TNF-alpha. *J. Immunol.* 171:6630-6639.

[146] Mishra, J., Ma, Q., Kelly, C., Mitsnefes, M., and Devarajan, P. 2006. Kidney NGAL is a novel early marker of acute injury following transplantation. *Pediatr. Nephrol.*

In: Acute Kidney Injury: Causes, Diagnosis and Treatments   ISBN: 978-1-61209-790-9
Editor: Jonathan D. Mendoza, pp. 141-166   © 2011 Nova Science Publishers, Inc.

Chapter IX

Sepsis: Acute Kidney Injury and β2-Adrenoceptor Therapy[*]

Akio Nakamura[†]

Department of Pediatrics, Teikyo University School of Medicine, 2-11-1, Kaga,
Itabashi-ku, Tokyo, Japan 173-8605

Abstract

Endotoxemia caused by Gram-negative bacteria can result in sepsis and organ dysfunction, which includes kidney injury and renal failure. The renal β_2-adrenoceptor (β_2-AR) system has an anti-inflammatory influence on the cytokine network during the course of immunologic responses. The previous reports indicated that the administration of β_2-AR agonists was found to attenuate the stimulation of renal TNF-α associated with lipopolysaccharide and Shiga toxin-2 of hemolytic uremic syndrome (HUS), which is considered to be a central mediator of the pathophysiologic changes. On the other hand, an altered expression and/or function of β_2-AR have been considered to be a pathogenetic factor in some disease states with inflammation; for example, heart failure and renal failure. These observations would suggest that blockade of functional β_2-AR activation might be associated with an increase risk for organ dysfunction following severe sepsis. In this chapter, we reviewed sepsis-induced renal injury and the genomic information to identify groups of patients with a high risk of developing sepsis-induced acute renal failure. In addition, we attempt to demonstrate a new insight into the immunological importance of β_2-AR activation in sepsis and an application of β_2-AR to septic renal failure and HUS. Furthermore, an *in vivo* β_2-AR gene therapy for the replacement of lost receptors as a consequence of sepsis was also described.

[*] A version of this chapter was also published in *Sepsis: Symptoms, Diagnosis and Treatment*, edited by Joseph R. Brown, published by Nova Science Publishers, Inc. It was submitted for appropriate modifications in an effort to encourage wider dissemination of research.
[†] E-mail: akio@med. teikyo-u. ac. jp , FAX: 03-3579-8212, TEL: 03-3964-1211 (ext. 7077)

Introduction

According to the 1992 Consensus Conference on definitions for sepsis and organ failure, sepsis is defined as a systemic inflammatory response (SIRS) associated with infection (Figure 1). Sepsis leads to the excessive production of proinflammatory cytokines, which are considered to contribute to the development of organ failure and tissue inflammation [1, 2]. This response is especially pertinent in acute inflammatory diseases, such as acute renal failure (ARF), as inflammatory mediators can cause a dose-related reversible response in target endothelial cells.

There is a growing body of evidence that the β_2-adrenoceptor (β_2-AR) system has an anti-inflammatory influence on the cytokine network during the course of immunologic responses. For example, β_2-AR agonists inhibit the renal production of inflammatory cytokines, such as tumour necrosis factor (TNF-α). Moreover, the administration of β_2AR agonists is found to attenuate TNF-α gene expression associated with Shiga toxin (Stx) of hemolytic uremic syndrome (HUS) [3]. Recently, we demonstrated that the application of adenoviral mediated β_2-AR gene delivery to enhance renal β_2-AR activity affords the kidney protection against endotoxin-induced ARF [4]. These observations would suggest a possibility that a level of functional β_2-AR activation might decide an increase risk for renal dysfunction following severe sepsis. Therefore, increased understanding of the immunologic basis of β_2-AR function in the kidney provides important new information relevant to the treatment of ARF in inflammatory diseases and potential applications of β_2-AR gene therapy in renal damage and inflammation associated with sepsis.

Sepsis-Induced Renal Injury

Acute Kidney Injury

Sepsis remains a worldwide problem and one that is associated with a high mortality rate. It is the leading cause of death in intensive care units (ICU) [5] and sepsis and its sequelae remains a major cause of ARF in both ICU and non-ICU [6]. ARF, recently renamed acute kidney injury (AKI), is a relatively frequent problem in patients with severe sepsis. Importantly, septic shock following surgery, trauma, burns, or severe infection was a common cause of ARF resulting in a high mortality rate [7]. It is recognized that severe sepsis results in excessive activation of inflammation and raised blood coagulation. In particular, endotoxemia caused by gram-negative bacteria can result in a systemic inflammatory response and organ dysfunction, which includes kidney ischemic and nephrotoxic damage [8, 9]. Pathological examination of the failing kidneys has revealed that inflammatory responses to sepsis resulted in the occurrence of focal necrosis of the proximal tubular epithelium, eosinophilic casts within proximal and distal tubules, and microthrombi in the glomerular capillaries [10]. Together these findings have implicated sepsis-induced inflammation, especially cytokines, in the pathogenesis of ARF.

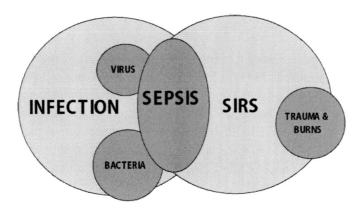

Figure 1. The definition of sepsis. Sepsis is defined as suspected or microbiologically proven infection together with SIRS.

Table 1. Positive association between sepsis with ARF or without ARF and polymorphisms

Genes	Allele	Illness/Ethnicity	Cases/Control subjects
TNF-α	TNF-α-308A	Sepsis/French whites	Septic shock/Healthy
		Septic shock	Survivors/non-Survivors
		ARF in neonate	ARF/non-ARF baby
		Post-operative sepsis/Taiwan Asian	Survivors/non-Survivors
		Dialysis-required ARF	Survivors/non-Survivors
TNF-β	TNF-β 252A homozygote	Post-operative sepsis/ German whites	Survivors/non-Survivors
IL-1ra	IL-raA2	Susceptibility to sepsis /German whites	Sepsis/Healthy
IL-6	IL-6-174C	ARF in neonate	ARF/non-ARF baby
IL-10	IL-10-592A	Sepsis	Survivors/non-Survivors
	IL-10-1082G	Dialysis-required ARF	Survivors/non-Survivors
HSP	HSP70-2+1267GG	ARF in neonate	ARF/non-ARF baby
	HSP70-2+1267AA	Septic shock	Sepsis/non-Sepsis
TLR4	Asp299Gly	Septic shock	Survivors/non-Survivors
		Septic shock	Septic shock/Healthy
CD14	CD14-159T	Septic shock/French whites	Sepsis/Healthy
		Septic shock/French whites	Survivors/non-Survivors

ARF:acute renal failure, HSP:heat shock protein, TLR:toll-like receptor.

Role of Cytokines in ARF

The role of pro-inflammatory cytokines in the development of endotoxin-mediated ARF has been increasingly recognized [11, 12]. TNF-α is a cytokine that initiates the inflammatory cascade that induces the production of numerous additional mediators associated with endothelial and tissue injury which comprise the multiple organ dysfunction syndrome [13-15]. Similarly, interleukin-10 (IL-10) is an important component of the anti-inflammatory cytokine network in sepsis which suppresses gene expression and synthesis of pro-inflammatory cytokines, such as TNF-α [16, 17]. These observations suggest that the balance between pro- and anti-inflammatory mediators plays an important role in the initiation and regulation of host inflammatory responses that determine the severity of acute illnesses such as ARF. Importantly, cytokines such as TNF-α, IL-1, IL-6, and IL-10 affect renal function in a variety of different ways [18]. High levels of these cytokines induce systemic hypotension which can lead to renal hypoperfusion; they directly influence renal hemodynamics by damaging glomerular endothelial and mesangial cells; they may induce the release and promote the effect of vasoactive mediators, such as endothelin, prostaglandins, and nitric oxide [19, 20]; finally, they may play a role in the initiation and progression of certain risk factors for ARF. In sepsis, cytokine release results in leukocyte activation along with the expression of adhesion molecules, oxygen-free radicals, arachidonic acid metabolites, platelet-activating factor, nitric oxide, endothelins, and heat shock proteins (HSP) [21,22]. Thus, it is this cytokine cascade that contributes to endothelial cell damage of the renal vasculature, leading to the development of ARF. Moreover, bacterial products can activate neutrophils within an already injured kidney [23], with IL-8 acting to recruit neutrophils to sites of inflammation [24]. Recently, human activated protein C, an endogenous protein that inhibits thrombosis and inflammation, decreased the relative risk of death in patients with severe sepsis [25]. However, it remains unclear which group of patients with sepsis benefit most from this therapy. Investigation into the specific genetic makeup may not only predict the risk of sepsis but may also to the development of organ dysfunction or ultimately death.

The Risk of ARF and Polymorphisms

Several studies have provided evidence supporting the view that genetic polymorphisms of cytokine-encoding genes can contribute to individual variance in inflammatory responses and they have postulated an association with risk for cytokine-mediated disorders, such as ARF (Table 1). It has been recognized that allelic polymorphisms in the promoter regions of cytokine genes regulate the expression of cytokines and may be of functional relevance. In particular, polymorphisms involving the promoter (5'-flanking) region of the TNF-α and IL-10 genes may affect transcriptional activity and thereby influence outcome in critically ill patients with ARF who require dialysis [26]. It has been reported that mortality is significantly higher in patients with the -308 G$\rightarrow$A polymorphism in the promoter region of the TNF-α gene, which was associated with higher levels of TNF-α production, and the -1082 G$\rightarrow$A polymorphism of the promoter region of the IL-10 gene, associated with lower levels of IL-10 production [26]. HSP72 plays a fundamental role in the ischemic tolerance of immature kidneys and protects premature babies against hypoxic renal injury [27, 28]. Fekete *et al.* [27] indicated that in low birth weight neonates carrying the HSP72 +1267GG genetic variation, which is associated with lower levels of HSP72 production, the risk of ARF was increased. Furthermore, they found that ARF risk was directly associated with high TNF-α producer and low IL-6 producer genotypes in preterm neonates [29]. On the other hand, several studies have found an association between the risk of sepsis and polymorphism of genes involved with the immune response genes; TNF-β gene variant [30], IL-1Ra allele-2 [31], IL-6-174C allele [32], IL-10-592A [33], CD14-159T [34], HSP70+2267AA [35], Toll like receptor(TLR)-4 Asp299Gly [36]. Polymorphism in these genes has been studied extensively and has been associated with adverse clinical outcomes among patients suffering from sepsis. However, these polymorphisms play in modulating susceptibility to or severity of ARF has not been investigated in sufficient depth to date.

Immunologic Effects of β₂-AR

Modulation of Immune Function

Sepsis involves activation of both the immune and the neuroendocrine systems. The modulation of immune function by catecholamines is pleiotypic and affects a range of cells in the immune system, including T cells, B cells, and NK cells [37]. In response to stress, norepinephrine and the related sympathetic catecholamine epinephrine are released into the blood-stream and in vitro they have been shown to alter several aspects of lymphocyte function, including inhibition of proliferation and differentiation [38], apoptosis [39], and interferon production in Th1 cells [40].

The β₂-ARs are distributed widely in vascular tissue and are the primary adrenergic receptor causing vasodilatation upon stimulation with endogenous catecholamines [41-43]. Furthermore, β₂-ARs are present on lymphocytes and are involved with the regulation of the immune responses. There is increasing evidence that activation of β₂-ARs can modulate the production of pro- and anti-inflammatory cytokines, such as TNF, IL-1, IL-6, IL-10, IL-12, in some tissues and organs [44-47]. We also demonstrated that in renal resident macrophage cells, the glomerular mesangial cells, and tubular epithelial cells and in brain astrocyte cells, the administration of β₂-AR agonists modulated the production and gene expression of TNF-α and IL-6 [45, 48]. An altered expression and function of the β₂-AR signal transduction mechanism in an organ is involved in the uncontrolled immune response that occurs during sepsis.

Anti-Inflammatory Effects in Sepsis

Bernardin et al. [49] showed that the activation of adenylate cyclase by β₂-AR was heterogeneously desensitized in peripheral blood mononuclear cells freshly isolated from septic patients. These observations would be compatible with the suggestion that abnormalities in the β₂-adrenergic control of organ function could be implicated in the pathogenesis of septic shock. β₂-AR agonists have been demonstrated to reduce both the increased permeability and the production of inflammatory mediators from endothelial cells [50, 51] and to prevent organ and tissue damage in response to an endotoxin challenge [3, 4]. Tighe et al. [52] have shown experimentally that in a porcine faecal peritonitis model of multi-organ failure, the administration of β_2-AR agonists reduces hepatic cellular injury during sepsis. Conversely, the β_2-AR antagonist, ICI 118551, enhanced the hepatic injury normally found during sepsis in the porcine model. These findings were supported by another report in which the β_2-AR agonist terbutaline was shown to attenuate the product of inflammatory cytokine mediators in the lungs and liver of sheep during endotoxic shock [30, 53]. On the other hand, in the kidney, it was found that the activation of β_2-ARs attenuated the production of TNF-α [4, 47] and suppressed kidney damage associated with the endotoxemia [54] and similarly the Stx-2 which causes HUS [3]. Endotoxin not only stimulates the production of cytokines but also the production of other mediators, such as histamine, leukotriene C and D, and prostaglandin D in human tissues. Importantly, β_2-AR agonists are able to suppress production of these mediators as well as cytokines [50, 55, 56]. Moreover, high levels of cyclic adenosine monophosphate (cAMP) in neutrophils caused by exposure to β_2-AR agonists can inhibit the generation of oxygen radicals [57]. It was further reported that a high level of cAMP in the endothelial cells was able to inhibit several key enzymes in the inflammatory pathway, leading to a reduced release of inflammatory mediators such as platelet-activating factor, histamine, and arachidonic acid derivatives [58]. Recent experiments indicated that the use of β_2-AR agonists had beneficial actions in chronic inflammatory diseases, including multiple sclerosis [59], rheumatoid arthritis [60], and hepatitis [61].

Intracellular Mechanisms

Intracellular signaling following β_2-AR activation is largely effected through a cAMP and protein kinase A (PKA) pathway. β_2-AR agonists activate their trimeric G protein-linked receptors to produce the stimulatory G protein (Gs) which stimulates adenylate cyclase to form cAMP and activate PKA. In the respiratory tract, cAMP induces airway relaxation through phosphorylation of muscle regulatory proteins and attenuation of cellular Ca^{2+} concentrations. Alternative cAMP-independent pathways have also been described involving activation of membrane maxi-K^+ channels and coupling through the inhibitory G protein (Gi) to the mitogen-activated protein kinase (MAPK) system.

The intracellular mechanisms by which activation of β_2-ARs inhibit inflammatory mediators has been examined by Tighe et al. [51]. In this study, they indicated that cAMP-PKA activation was involved in activating gene transcription agents to produce anti-inflammatory proteins such as IL-10. Moreover, PKA inhibited phospholipase C and MAPK to determine the production of pro-inflammatory cytokines. Additionally, van der Poll et al. [62] indicated that pre-exposure of healthy humans to a constant infusion of epinephrine before injection of endotoxin attenuates the production of the pro-inflammatory cytokine TNF-α and simultaneously potentiates the production of the anti-inflammatory cytokine IL-10 through the adenylate cyclase-cAMP-PKA pathway [63, 64]. Furthermore, Panina-Bordignon et al. [65] presented evidence that β_2-AR agonists inhibited IL-12 production by human monocytes in response to lipopolysaccharide (LPS). The β_2-AR mediated inhibition of IL-12 correlated with β_2-AR stimulation and with increased levels of intracellular cAMP. Taken together, it is recognized that the cAMP-PKA pathway plays a critical role in the regulation of inflammatory cytokine production via β_2-AR activation.

Kidney and β_2-AR System

β_2-AR

β-AR belongs to a large family of the G-protein-coupled receptors that are characterized by seven transmembrane helices. Three subtypes of β-ARs (β_1-AR, β_2-AR, β_3-AR) are detected in the mammalian tissues. Molecular biological cloning approaches showed that β_2-AR gene is an intronless single gene coding 413 amino acid and is located on chromosome 5q31-33. β_2-ARs are involved in fundamental processes such as cell growth, differentiation, and metabolism and play important roles in cardiovascular, respiratory, metabolic, reproductive and central nervous system functions (Table 2). The β_2-ARs are found throughout the body including the heart, lung, blood vessels, lymphocyte and kidneys. In the heart, β_2-ARs have been localized to the ventricular walls where they primarily determine ventricular contractility. In the respiratory tract, the β_2-ARs are the predominant subtype in all segments but the β_2-AR-mediated adenylate cyclase response is tissue-dependent, with higher activity being present in the tracheal membranes than the bronchial or pulmonary segments. The β_2-ARs are also distributed widely in vascular tissue and are the primary adrenergic receptor causing vasodilatation upon stimulation with endogenous catecholamines. In clinical medicine, β_2-AR agonists are standard agents in the treatment of bronchial asthma and chronic bronchitis. A majority of β_2–AR agonists is eliminated via the kidneys as an unchanged substance. It is likely that such agents will exert pharmacological effects during their passage through the nephron. However, these pharmacological effects have, to our knowledge, not been taken into consideration when using these compounds in clinical practice because a role of β_2–AR in the regulation of renal function remains unclear.

Renal β_2–AR Pharmacology

The β-ARs are located in the kidneys [66-68] and the receptors are known to participate in the regulation of glomerular filtration rate (GFR), sodium reabsorption, acid-base balance and renin secretion [69]. Immunoreactivity for β_1-ARs was found in mesangial cells, juxtaglomerular granular cells, the macula densa epithelium, proximal and distal tubular segments, and acid-secreting type A intercalated cells of the cortical and medullary collecting ducts. On the other hand, β_2-ARs were predominantly localized in the apical and subapical compartment of proximal and, to a lesser extent, distal tubular epithelia [69]. This anatomic location provides evidence for a role of β_2-ARs in the control of renal tubular function. It has been reported that β_2-AR activation enhances sodium reabsorption through increased renal epithelial sodium channel (ENaC) activity [70-72]. In addition, the presence of functional β_2-AR in cultured rat proximal tubule epithelial cells was demonstrated by the observation that

β_2-AR activation resulted in increases in Sodium-Potassium-adenosine triphosphatase (Na-K-ATPase) activity and transcellular sodium transport as a consequence of increased apical sodium entry [73].

Furthermore, Singh and Linas[74] found that β_2-AR-mediated increases in Na-K-ATPase activity and sodium flux were transduced by protein kinase C (PKC), not PKA, acting to increase apical Na entry. In an *in vivo* study, Hashimoto *et al.* [75] indicated that β_2-AR activation produced a decrease in urine flow, free water and osmolar clearance and also excretion of electrolytes in rat and dog renal tubules. In addition, they showed that renal blood flow and GFR were reduced by β_2-AR agonists with the concomitant fall of systemic blood pressure [75]. Boivin *et al.* [69] reported that there was a high density of β_2-ARs in the membranes of smooth muscle cells from renal arteries. Administration of β_2-AR agonists had no effect on blood coagulation or hemolysis but inhibited the edema and increase in permeability of blood vessels induced by acetic acid [75]. Thus, the β_2- adrenergic system has the ability to modulate both the renal vasculature and renal tubule solute and water transport.

Table 2. Effects of β_2 adrenoceptor agonist

System	adrenoceptor type	Response to stimulation
Heart	$\beta 1 \beta 2$	Tachycardia
	$\beta 1$	Contraction
Bronchus	$\beta 2$	Dilatation
Brain	$\beta 1 \beta 2$	?
Gut	$\beta 1$	Relaxation
	$\beta 3$	
Metabolism	$\beta 2$	Inhibition (Insulin secretion)
	$\beta 3$	Lipolysis
Vessel	$\beta 1$	Dilatation (Coronary arteries)
	$\beta 2$	Dilatation (Renal arteries)
Kidney	$\beta 1$	Stimulation (Renin secretion)
	$\beta 2$	Sodium reabsorption

Defense Mechanisms for Septic ARF

(1) Inhibition of renal TNF-α production

In many types of renal glomerulonephritis, macrophages infiltrate into the glomerulus and interstitium and this has been taken as being the initial step in inducing renal damage [76]. Furthermore, it has been reported that macrophages are involved in the development of interstitial nephritis and obstructive uropathy [77]. Although the mechanisms mediating the macrophage-induced renal damage remains unclear, the pathophysiological developments in these renal diseases are associated with raised TNF-α [76] which plays a role in ischemic and toxic chemical injury within renal tissue [78]. Thus, there is a strong possibility that renal TNF-α generation is one of the most important factors in the pathophysiology of renal disease and injury. Previous investigators [47] have reported that elevation of intracellular cAMP is associated with the suppression of macrophage activation and cytokine production. Our own studies in the kidney also demonstrated that activation of the cAMP signaling pathway by means of β_2-AR agonists down-regulated TNF-α gene expression using renal resident macrophage cells exposed to endotoxin[80]. Consequently, the renal β_2-AR system was able to modify the inflammatory responses initiated in sepsis-induced renal injury through the inhibition of renal TNF-α generation.

(2) Modulation of IL-6

Amongst these pro-inflammatory cytokines, IL-6 is a pleiotropic cytokine which is involved in inflammatory and immune responses, acute phase reactions and hematopoiesis. At the level of the kidney, IL-6 is a key factor in mediating various components of the immune and inflammatory response [81]. There is increasing evidence that activation of β_2-ARs can modulate the production of LPS-induced inflammatory cytokines. However, the action of β_2-AR stimulation on IL-6 production is quite controversial. Liao et al. [46] observed that β_2-AR mediated processes increased LPS-induced IL-6 production in liver cells, while Maimone et al. [82] reported that exposure of astrocytes to norepinephrine elevated IL-6 which was mediated predominantly by β_2-AR and the activation of adenylate cyclase. It is recognized that intracellular cAMP plays an important role in the stimulation of IL-6 gene expression [83] and it has been suggested that raised IL-6 production due to β_2-AR activation is mediated through the cAMP pathway. On the other hand, Straub et al. [84] demonstrated that isoproterenol inhibited IL-6 secretion in the spleen, while our own studies also indicated an inhibitory effect of β_2-AR activation following LPS-induced IL-6 gene transcription in rat astrocytes [85]. Furthermore, in an in vivo study, epinephrine infusion into human subjects did not affect IL-6 production following an LPS challenge [62]. These findings suggest that factors and/or regulatory mechanisms other than the cAMP pathway contribute to β_2-AR mediated IL-6 production. Therefore, using renal resident macrophage cells treated with endotoxin, LPS, and β_2-AR agonist, terbutaline, we investigated the intracellular mechanisms in up-regulating or down-regulating IL-6 production [70].

The results from this experiment, terbutaline at high concentrations (10^{-6}M) significantly up-regulated IL-6 by approximately 25% (P < 0. 05), whereas at a lower concentration (10^{-8}M), it down-regulated IL-6 production by 42% (P < 0. 05). Terbutaline (10^{-8}M and 10^{-6}M) caused a concentration and time-dependent stimulation of cAMP (P<0. 05) and a time-dependent decrease in MAPK activity (P<0. 05) and TNF-α production (P<0. 05).

Following the addition of a cAMP inhibitor, IL-6 promoter activity was correlated with TNF-α levels and MAPK activity. The terbutaline-induced down-regulation of IL-6 gene production was mediated by an inhibitory effect of terbutaline on TNF-α, which was exerted through the MAPK and cAMP pathways, whereas the up-regulation appeared to be due to a direct action of intracellular cAMP. Therefore, the modulation of endotoxin-induced IL-6 levels by β_2-ARs depends on the balance between a direct effect of cAMP as a stimulator of IL-6 and an indirect action of TNF-α as a suppresser of IL-6 through cAMP and/or MAPK (p42/p44) pathways.

(3) Inhibition of apoptosis

HUS is characterized by renal failure, thrombocytopenia and hemolytic anemia and is often induced by Stx producing strains of *Escherichia coli* [86, 87]. The most extensive tissue damage in HUS occurs in the kidney and reports have indicated that renal tubular impairment is a contributor to the development of HUS [88, 89]. Stx induces an apoptotic signal transduction cascade associated with enhanced expression of Bax in epithelial cells and the Stx-stimulated cell death was blocked by overexpression of Bcl-2 [90, 91]. Zhu et al. [92] observed that the β_2-AR agonist, clenbuterol, not only increased Bcl-2 expression but also decreased Bax expression in a rat model of forebrain ischemia. These findings suggested the possibility that β_2-AR activation could have a major anti-apoptotic action. To provide further support for this view, we investigated the molecular mechanisms underlying the action of β_2-AR stimulation on Stx-induced apoptosis [93]. Apoptosis is regulated by several pathways, such as caspases, MAPK and cAMP-PKA cascade. This experiment focused on the effect of β_2-AR activation on Stx2-induced apoptosis in renal tubular cells and the contribution of these signaling pathways.

Cultured human adenocarcinoma-derived renal tubular cells (ACHN) were exposed to Stx (64 pg/mL) for 2–24 hr following the addition of the β_2-AR agonist (terbutaline) to the incubation medium. Stx-induced apoptosis and its amelioration by β_2-AR activation was confirmed using DNA degradation assays and by flow cytometry for annexin V, mitochondrial membrane potential and caspase (-3 and -7) activity. Exposure of cells to Stx for 24 hr increased the DNA fragmentation to 11. 6±0. 9%, compared to 3. 3±0. 2% in control cells ($P<0. 05$) but was decreased to approximately 5–7% ($P<0. 05$) in the presence of terbutaline. Furthermore, Stx-stimulated apoptosis, detected by TUNEL, annexin V and mitochondrial potential, was inhibited by terbutaline ($P<0. 05$) which was prevented by cAMP-PKA inhibitors and a β_2-AR antagonist. However, inhibition of Stx-mediated caspase activity by terbutaline was partially blocked by cAMP-PKA inhibitors. On the other hand, p38MAPK inhibition by terbutaline prevented Stx-induced apoptosis and caspase activity through a cAMP-independent pathway via β_2-AR. These data indicate that β_2-AR activation can inhibit Stx-induced apoptosis of the cells, which may be caused by a reduction in caspase activity through cAMP-PKA activation and the p38MAPK pathway (Figure 2).

(4) Modulation of innate immunity

LPS is sensed by LPS-binding protein (LBP), CD14, and toll-like receptor 4 (TLR4). CD14/ TLR4 complexes are the primary signaling receptor for gram-negative bacterial LPS [94]. When presented to CD14 by LBP, LPS is delivered to high-affinity transmembrane receptor such as TLR4 [95], leading to production of TNF-α [96]. Thus, CD14 and TLR4 are critical for LPS-mediated production of TNF- α. Injection of LPS reproduces many of the manifestations of sepsis and organ dysfunction, including kidney damage and renal failure [9]. The pathological mechanisms responsible for this renal dysfunction involve several mediators, and an important class is the early proinflammatory cytokines, such as TNF-α [78, 79]. Cunningham et al. [97] have showed that mice deficient in tumour necrosis factor receptor 1 (TNFR1) are resistant to LPS-induced ARF, and that TNFR1 mediates LPS-induced ARF within the kidney. Therefore, these evidences suggest a possibility that activation of β₂-AR signaling pathway could attenuate renal TNF-α production through CD14 and TLR4-dependent mechanisms, which, in turn, contributes to the protection against LPS-induced ARF. Recently, we clarified the importance of functional β₂-AR in regulating innate immunity in LPS-induced ARF [98]. In the animal experiment, rats were challenged with LPS, and the role of β₂-AR-mediated intrarenal cAMP in the regulation of CD14-TLR4-TNF-α signaling pathway in the kidney was determined using co-administration with β₂-AR antagonist ICI118, 551.

Figure 2 depicts these findings and summarizes the known effects of LPS and Stx and the possible interaction with β₂-AR signaling pathway.

Strategy for Septic ARF

β₂-AR Agonists

(1) Endotoxin-induced sepsis

Cytokines play an important role in pathogenesis of endotoxin-induced ARF. Some studies indicated that β₂-AR activation regulated TNF-α and IL-6 production in cultured cells stimulated by endotoxin. In liver cells, Liao *et al.* [46] documented that β₂-AR -mediated processes were able to regulate TNF- α and IL-6 production. Severn *et al.* [47] demonstrated suppression of TNF-α production by isoproterenol in cultured human blood cells stimulated by LPS, which was mediated by increased intracellular cAMP levels. Hetier *et al.* [48] investigated the regulation of TNF- α gene expression in the microglia cells upon stimulation with LPS, and observed that isoproterenol, via an action at β₂-AR, was able to influence the regulatory processes of TNF- α gene expression. In the kidney, we have reported that LPS-stimulated TNF- α and IL-6 gene transcription, mRNA accumulation and protein levels were suppressed by β₂-AR activation with terbutaline using cultured renal resident macrophage cells [80] and mesangial cells [45,99].

There is also *in vivo* evidence that β₂-AR agonists can modulate the production of TNF-α and IL-6 in some tissues and organs under the state of endotoxemia. Previously, we investigated whether, *in vivo*, the administration of β₂-AR agonists regulate renal TNF- α and IL-6 mRNA following LPS stimulation to cause endotoxaemia [100]. In this experiment, 4-

week-old Wistar rats pre-treated with the β_2-AR agonist terbutaline or formoterol, and/or the β-AR and β_2-AR antagonists (propanolol, ICI118,551), were injected with LPS (1 mg i. p.), and then 2, 4 or 6 h later, kidneys (cortex, medulla), spleen, thymus and plasma were assayed TNF-α and IL-6 mRNA levels and their respective protein release. The results indicated that administration of β_2-AR agonists suppressed TNF-α mRNA expression in the whole kidney, by 61% ($P<0. 05$), as well as plasma, spleen and thymus TNF-α protein and mRNA expression 2 h after injection of LPS. On the other hand, although IL-6 levels in plasma, spleen and thymus mRNA expression were suppressed significantly by administration of β_2-AR agonists, the basal- and LPS-induced IL-6 mRNA levels in the whole kidney were increased 1. 6- and 1. 2-fold ($P<0. 05$), respectively, by treatment with β_2-AR agonists. These findings suggest the existence of tissue specific regulation of IL-6 production in the kidney by β_2-AR activation.

(2) HUS

As described previously, Stx-producing *Escherichia coli* are responsible for some cases of HUS [86, 87]. There are two forms of Stx and they are also known as verocytotoxins, Stx1 and Stx2. It has been reported that induction of the globotriaosyleramide (Gb3) receptor, known to be the functional receptor for Stx, is one mechanism by which inflammatory mediators increase susceptibility to Stx [101]. The major pathogenesis of HUS has been ascribed to initial endothelial and vascular damage. However, evidence has been reported from some studies in human, of primary renal tubular cell damage in HUS [89]. The receptor sites for Stx binding in normal kidney sections are most prominent in renal cortical tubules [89,102], probably in the distal tubule. Renal biopsy studies early in the course of HUS have suggested a direct action on the proximal tubules while cultured epithelial cells from this region express very high levels of Gb3 [90,103]. These reports imply that renal tubular impairment contributes to the development of HUS.

Exposure of renal tubular epithelial cells to Stx causes cytotoxicity, and the potency of this toxin is enhanced in the presence of TNF-α [88]. It has been shown that Stx induces TNF-α production and that activation of β_2-ARs downregulates TNF-α. However, little was known about the signaling pathway by which β_2-AR agonists suppress the Stx-induced TNF-α gene transcription in the renal tubular cells. Previously, we investigated that the possible signaling components involved in this pathway [3]. In this experiment, MAPK, activating protein-1 (AP-1), and nuclear factor-κB (NFκ-B) were measured to evaluate the regulatory mechanisms involved in TNF-α gene transcription in ACHN exposed to Stx in the presence or absence of a β_2-AR agonist. Stx (4 pg/ml) stimulated MAPK (p42/p44, p38) and AP-1 and increased TNF-α promoter activity by 2. 4-fold. The increase in TNF-α was attenuated by both a p42/p44 inhibitor, PD098059 (10^{-6} M), and a p38 inhibitor, SB203580 (10^{-6} M), and AP-1—binding activity was inhibited by PD098059. Terbutaline (10^{-6} M to 10^{-8} M) suppressed MAPK (p42/p44, p38), NF-κB (p50, p65), and TNF-α promoter activity in a dose-dependent way that was prevented by the β_2-AR antagonist, ICI118,551. However, inhibition of MAPK (p42/p44) and TNF-α promoter activity was partially prevented by the cAMP-protein kinase (PKA) inhibitors, H-89 (5 x 10^{-6} M) and KT5720 (10^{-5} M), whereas the suppression of p38 MAPK or NF-κB (p50) was not blocked by these inhibitors. The suppression of NF-κB (p65) was completely overcome by H-89 or KT5720. Consequently, the downregulation of TNF-α transcription by terbutaline was mediated by an inhibitory effect of β₂-AR activation on MAPK (p42/p44, p38) and NF-κB p50/p65), which were exerted through a cAMP-PKA pathway and a cAMP-independent mechanism (Figure 2).

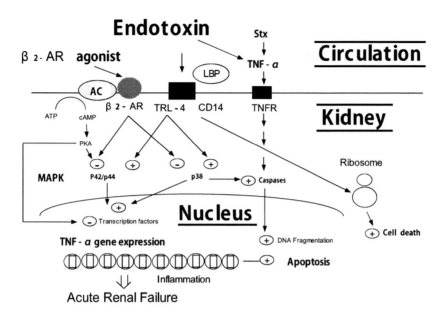

Figure 2. Proposed model of pathways mediating TNF-α production and apoptosis in renal cells exposed to endotoxin, Stx and/or β₂-adrenoceptor (β₂-AR) agonists. Endotoxin sensed by LBP initiates intracellular signaling events via CD14 and TLR-4 in the kidney. The CD14 and TLR-4 complexes could result in the stimulation of renal TNF-α production through the activation of transcription factors (AP-1, NF-κB) via MAPK signaling cascades. Stx also stimulates TNF-α gene expression through these signaling cascades and activated caspase cascade (caspase-3), thereby signaling cells to undergo apoptosis. On the other hand, β₂-ARs couple to adenylate cyclases (AC) to raise intracellular level of cAMP-PKA, which inhibits TLR4-CD14-TNF-α signaling cascades, p42/p44 MAPK and caspases activation. Moreover, β₂-AR activation suppresses p38 MAPK activity with subsequent caspase-3 inhibition through a cAMP-independent mechanism. Importantly, β₂-AR activation inhibits the renal TNF-α–induced inflammation and apoptosis associated with endotoxin and Stx, which, in turn, could result in ARF. +: activation, - :inhibition.

β₂-AR Gene Therapy

(1) Contribution of β₂-AR gene delivery to renal physiology

For the purpose of activation and restoration of β₂-AR function, drugs targeting β₂-AR signaling, including β₂-AR agonists, may be used as a first-line approach for therapy. However, administration of β₂-AR agonists to regulate β₂-AR function has an inherently limited efficacy, partly because of the down-regulation and desensitization of β₂-ARs [99]. On the other hand, *in vivo* gene therapy using adenoviral constructs containing the β₂-AR gene has been demonstrated to be an efficient and reproducible global transgene delivery system which results in long term expression in the organ as has been reported in the myocardium [105]. Therefore, the application of adenoviral mediated β₂-AR gene delivery to elevate β₂-AR density and prevent desensitization would be an attractive option whereby β₂-

ARs could be active over a prolonged period. With this in mind we utilized adenoviral-mediated β_2-AR gene delivery to investigate whether over-expression of β_2-AR could alter both biochemical and *in vivo* renal function and to test the hypothesis that the β_2-AR gene delivery affords the kidney protection against endotoxin-induced ARF [4]. As a construction of recombinant adenovirus, the human β_2-AR expressing adenovirus (Adeno-β_2-AR) and the cytoplasmic β-galactosidase expressing adenovirus (Adeno-LacZ) as a control were used in the study. These adenoviruses were a replication-deficient first-generation type V adenovirus with deletions of the E1 gene (Figure 3). These viruses were injected into the right kidney of rats using a 25-gauge needle attached to a 1ml syringe.

To test how long β_2–AR transgene over expression was supported in the renal tissue, β–AR density levels were measured in the right and left kidneys during a 5 wk period after intraparenchymal gene delivery. There was a sharp increase in β–AR density level 2 wks after intraparenchymal Adeno-β_2–AR gene delivery (10^9 total viral particles:t. v. p) in the right kidney, which was sustained until the 4 wk time-point. Furthermore, measurable β–AR over expression was also observed in the contra-lateral left kidney, which was elevated at 2 wks after the gene delivery. β–AR density in the right and left kidneys after intraparenchymal Adeno- LacZ gene delivery (10^9 t. v. p) was unaltered over this timeframe.

The time course of glomerular filtration rate (GFR:ml/min/100g body weight) after delivery of various doses of Adeno-β_2–AR was investigated. Although there was a significant increase (P<0. 05) in GFR 2wks after intraparenchymal delivery of Adeno-β_2–AR (10^9t. v. p), GFR levels at 1, 3, and 4wks after delivery of Adeno-β_2–AR (10^{8-9}t. v. p) were not changed compared to those in Adeno- LacZ treated rats. In contrast, the higher dose of 10^{10}t. v. p Adeno-β_2–AR produced a diminished GFR with advancing age. The changes in time course of FENa or FEK (%) following various doses of Adeno-β_2–AR were also measured over this timeframe. There was a significant decrease in FENa (P<0.05) 1-2wks after intraparenchymal delivery of Adeno-β_2–AR(10^{8-9}t. v. p), while at 3 and 4wks after delivery of Adeno-β_2–AR (10^{8-9}t. v. p) it was not different from that in Adeno- LacZ treated rats. FEK levels after delivery of Adeno-β_2–AR (10^{8-9}t. v. p) were unchanged compared to those in Adeno- LacZ treated rats while there was a significant increase in FEK 3-4wks after intraparenchymal delivery of the higher dose of Adeno-β_2–AR (10^{10}t. v. p). These results indicated that GFR, FENa, and FEK became stable approximately 3-4 wks after the delivery of Adeno-β_2–AR (10^{8-9}t. v. p). Furthermore, Adeno- β_2–AR (10^9 t. v. p) did not change weight, Blood Pressure (BP) or Heart Rate compared with those of physiological saline (PBS) treated rats without adenovirus delivery. This suggested the safety of Adeno- β_2–AR (10^9 t. v. p) delivery.

(2) Effects of β_2–AR gene therapy on septic ARF

These effects were investigated using intraperitoneal injection of LPS (5mg/kg) to induce renal failure in control and Adeno-β_2–AR treated rats. Control rats of this experiment were injected intraperitoneally with an equal volume of PBS. The β_2-AR antagonist ICI 118,551 was given intraperitoneally 2 h before an injection of the LPS or PBS. The experiment was performed on the 25th day after the delivery of 10^9 t. v. p of Adeno-β_2–AR, which was chosen as the therapeutic dose [4]. It can be seen in Figure 4 that GFR in the Adeno-β_2–AR treated rats was not changed 24h after the injection of LPS while in the control rats it was significantly (P<0. 05) depressed by the LPS challenge. The addition of the antagonist, ICI

118,551 blocked the ability of the Adeno-β_2–AR treated rats to maintain GFR, suggesting that constitutive β_2–AR activity plays an important role in preserving renal function against the endotoxin. Figure 5 indicated that β_2–AR density measured in the right kidney from control rats was significantly (P<0. 05) depressed 24 h after the LPS challenge. The renal β_2–AR density in Adeno-β_2–AR treated rats, although higher than the control rats, was also decreased by the injection of LPS (P<0. 05). Besides kidney, the lung β_2–AR levels were also depressed by the treatments with LPS (Figure 5). On the other hand, renal cAMP content (of both right and left kidneys) was depressed (P<0. 05) by the LPS challenge in the control rats but not in the Adeno-β_2–AR treated rats. The responses in renal cAMP level induced by the LPS in both groups correlated with the changes in renal β–AR density.

Recombinant Adenoviral Constructs

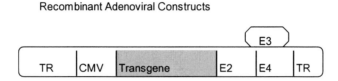

Figure 3. The human β_2-AR expressing adenovirus (Adeno-β_2-AR) and the cytoplasmic β-galactosidase expressing adenovirus (Adeno-LacZ) as a control

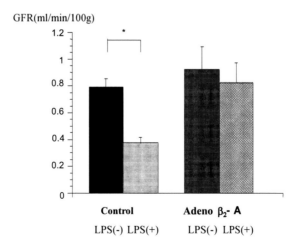

Figure 4. Rescue of endotoxin-induced renal dysfunction in the Adeno-β_2-AR rats. GFR (ml/min per 100 g body weight) levels in rats treated with PBS (control) or Adeno-β_2-AR were estimated 24h after LPS (5 mg/kg intraperitoneally) injection. Data are mean ± SE. *P<0. 05 *versus* PBS or Adeno-β_2-AR rats without LPS treatment. n = 5 to 8.

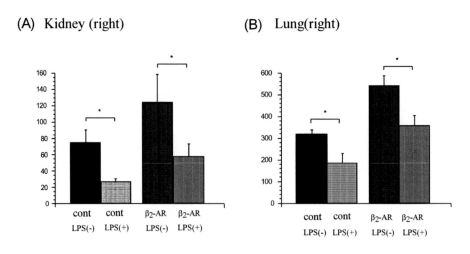

(A) Kidney (right)   (B) Lung(right)

β2-adrenoceptor density
(f mol/mg membrane protein)

Figure 5. β_2-AR density levels of the right kidney(A) and the right lung (B) in rats treated with PBS (control) or Adeno-β_2-AR were estimated 24h after LPS (5 mg/kg intraperitoneally) injection. Data are mean ± SE. *P<0. 05 *versus* PBS or Adeno-β_2-AR rats without LPS treatment. n =6 to 8.

From these findings, we found that renal over expression of β_2–ARs using gene transfer with Adeno-β_2–AR was effective in preventing endotoxin-induced renal injury. This finding was intriguing in that the sepsis induced renal failure occurred with the decreases in β_2-AR density and cAMP activity, which suggested an impaired renal β_2–AR signaling system. Thus, the delivery of Adeno-β_2-AR gene could be a potential novel therapeutic strategy for treatment of ARF associated with sepsis. It is likely that this protective effect of β_2-AR activation is exerted through the intracellular cAMP-PKA pathway as previous studies reported found that cAMP-PKA activation was necessary to prevent the development of ARF [106]. Indeed, it was reported that the fall in renal cAMP level was correlated with the depression in GFR caused by the LPS challenge [107].

(3) Optional route of administration and safety
In clinical trials with adenoviral vectors, route-dependent efficacy of gene therapy has been a significant concern [108]. Generally, the direct injection into the target organ is more efficacious than systemic administration, via intravenous or intramuscular routes. However, gene therapy aimed to overcome systemic inflammation, for example as occurs in sepsis, requires a suitable injection route for the viral gene vector, such that it can effectively incorporate into the major target organs of sepsis, the kidney, lung, liver, and heart. An additional consideration of gene therapy using adenoviral vectors is the potential toxicity, which may cause inflammation on the tissues [109]. Therefore, high transduction rates, bio-safety of the gene product and minimally invasive administration are required to ensure an optimal route of gene delivery for a successful therapeutic strategy for sepsis.

The subcutaneous route can be used as it does not require particular techniques or surgical manipulation and therefore it may be an option as a route of delivery of the vector and could be clinically relevant. However, it remains unclear whether subcutaneous delivery of Adeno-β_2-AR might be effective in providing sustained and therapeutic levels of the transgene in the target organs. Furthermore, viral vectors have some negative characteristics, mainly that they can trigger inflammatory and immune responses with the possibility that adenovirus gene therapy may worsen the outcome of sepsis. With this in mind, we have undertaken the experiment [110] to explore whether the utilization of the subcutaneous injection technique could potentiate the β_2-AR signaling systems in the kidney and at the same time to test the safety of gene product. Furthermore, we have sought to evaluate its efficacy in preventing endotoxin-induced renal dysfunction.

The results from this experiment demonstrated that Adeno-β_2-AR (10^{10} t. v. p) delivery via the subcutaneous route was effective in providing sustained levels of the transgene in the target organ, of at least a doubling of the endogenous content for at least three weeks. Interestingly, a similar magnitude and pattern of changes in adrenoceptor content were also observed in the lung but to a lesser extent in the liver and heart. Importantly, it was evident from the physiological parameters, which is body weight, BP and plasma biochemistry that these were very comparable in the control and viral vector treated groups of rats and suggested that the vector had no untoward effect at least in the three week time frame. Moreover, the histological evaluation of the kidney, lung, liver, and heart showed that a 10^{10} t. v. p dose of Adeno-β_2-AR did not produce any evidence of cellular deterioration or toxicity using this adenoviral approach. It has been reported that adenoviral gene therapy induced a proinflammatory response in the lung and liver, characterized by increased TNF-α expression [111, 112]. However, under the conditions of this study there was no elevation in TNF-α mRNA levels as a consequence of the Adeno-β_2-AR administration. Furthermore, this study showed that the plasma cytokine levels were not increased in the Adeno-β_2-AR treated rats. Together, these findings provide support for the view that Adeno-β_2-AR (10^{10} t. v. p) delivery via the subcutaneous route did not initiate any inflammatory responses at least over the three week period of observation. Nevertheless, the possibility remains that over a longer time frame integrating adenoviral vectors into the body might carry a greater risk of malignancy due to their ability to randomly integrate into the target genomes. An important outcome is that further basic study will be required to improve and further evaluate the technical aspects of the gene therapy using adenoviral vectors.

(4) Other gene therapies to sepsis

Some investigators have evaluated the effect of adenoviral vector gene transfer in animal models to overcome the consequences of sepsis. Alexander et al. [113] demonstrated that adenoviral gene transfer of human bactericidal/permeability increasing protein (BPI) inhibited the effect of a non lethal dose of LPS on cytokine responses and improved the survival of mice subject to lethal septic shock. On the basis of these results, they suggested that human BPI gene transfer had the potential of being used as a therapeutic agent for septic conditions. In addition, Minter et al. [114] reported that adenoviral expression of the anti-inflammatory cytokine IL-10 could be successfully used in the treatment of two acute inflammatory disease situations, for example, necrotizing pancreatitis and multisystem organ failure. However, whether these in vivo gene therapies prevented the progression of organ dysfunction associated with endotoxemia remains unclear. It was of concern that although administration of these genes effectively supported organ functions, these gene therapies were not able to survive all of the endotoxemic animals. Therefore, the gene therapy and adjuvant supportive cares therapy and early administration of empirical antibiotic therapy may be also required to improve the survival of the patients with sepsis [115].

Conclusion

Sepsis caused by bacteria and toxin is a common cause of ARF resulting in a high mortality rate in children. Cytokine production and release, HSP expression, nitric oxide synthesis activity, coagulation factors or factors of the innate immune system-like defenses involved in inflammation, contribute to a wide range of clinical manifestations of an inflammatory disease. Interestingly, functional β_2-AR activation is also involved in SIRS associated with endotoxemia and HUS and contributes to the treatment of some inflammatory diseases, including sepsis. Importantly, it was reported that cAMP-PKA activation is a central component in the protection against endotoxin-induced ARF. The β_2-AR activation could potentially be an important genetic factor pre-determining the degree of pathobiology of endotoxin-induced ARF and Stx-induced HUS. Importantly, constitutive β_2-AR activation after the Adeno-β_2-AR gene delivery was able to protect renal function through several mechanisms, including the cAMP-PKA pathway. The model presented herein is of *in vivo* gene transfer of Adeno-β_2–AR into the kidney, which has been demonstrated to be an efficient and reproducible global delivery of transgene to the renal glomeruli and tubular epithelial cells of the rat (Figure 6). In this model, we present novel findings indicating that the delivery of Adeno-β_2-AR gene is a potential novel therapeutic strategy for treatment of ARF associated with sepsis. Together, these findings suggest that functional β_2-AR activation may be a potential prophylactic/therapeutic approach in patients at high risk of developing ARF or patients who suffer sepsis but have not yet developed renal failure.

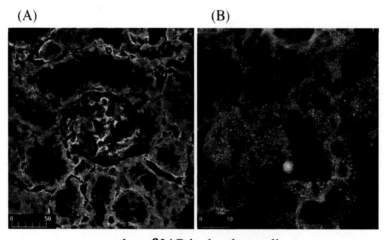

(A)   (B)

adeno-β2AR in the glomeruli

Figure 6. Immunohistochemical detection of β_2-AR expressed in the right kidney 4 wk after intraparenchymal injection (10^9 t. v. p.) of Adeno-β_2-AR–treated rats. β_2-AR was not only expressed in renal tubules (A: Scale bars: 50 μm) but also in glomeruli (B: Scale bars: 10 μm). White signals in the cells indicate β_2-AR expression.

Acknowledgements

I am very grateful for support from a Grant-in-Aid for Scientific Research from the Ministry of Education, Sports, Science and Technology, Japan (17590845) and Kawano Masanori Memorial Foundation for Promotion of Pediatrics. I thank Prof. E.J. Johns. Department of Physiology, University of Cork, Ireland, for critical review of the manuscript and suggestions and Mrs. Kumiko Kurosaki for technical support.

References

[1] Christenson, J. T., Sigurdsson, G. H., Mousawi, M. & Owunwanne, A. (1987). Use of indium-111 oscine to study the effects of terbutaline on pulmonary and hepatic plateletsequestration in endotoxin shock. *Am. J. Physiol. Imaging, 2,* 186-191.

[2] Gluser, M. P., Zanetti, G., Baumgartner, J. D. & Cohen, J. (1991). Septic shock: pathogenesis. *Lancet, 338,* 732-736.

[3] Nakamura, A., Johns, E. J., Imaizumi, A., Yanagawa, Y. & Kohsaka, T. (2001). Activation of β-adrenoceptor prevents shiga toxin-induced tumour necrosis factor production. *J. Am. Soc. Nephrol, 12,* 2288-2299.

[4] Nakamura, A., Imaizumi, A., Yanagawa, Y., Kohsaka, T. & Johns, E. J. (2004). β_2-Adrenoceptor activation attenuates endotoxin-induced acute renal failure. *J. Am. Soc. Nephrol, 15,* 316–325.

[5] Collins, F. S. (1999). Shattuck lecture: medical and societal consequences of the Human Genome Project. *N. Engl. J. Med, 341,* 28-37.

[6] Liano, F., Junco, E., Madero, R., Pascual, J. & Verde, E. (1998). The spectrum of acute renal failure in the intensive care unit compared with that seen in other settings. The Madrid Acute renal Failure Study Group. *Kidney Int., 66,* S16-S24.

[7] Schor, N. (2002). Acute renal failure and the sepsis syndrome. *Kidney Int., 61,* 764-776.

[8] Kikeri, D., Pennel, J. P., Hwang, K. H., Jakob, J. I., Richman, A. V. & Bourgigne, J. J. (1986). Endotoxemic acute renal failure in awake rats. *Am. J. Physiol, 250,* F1098-F1106.

[9] Zager, R. A. (1986). Escherichia coli endotoxin injections potentiate experimental ischemic renal injury. *Am. J. Physiol, 251,* F988-F994.

[10] Kaplan, S. L. (1998). Bacteremia and septic shock in *Textbook of Pediatric Infectious Diseases, (4).* Edited by Feigin, R. D. & Cherry, J. D. Philadelphia, WB Saunders, 807-820.

[11] Wiecek, A., Zeier, M. & Ritz, E. (1994). Role of infection in the genesis of acute renal failure. *Nephrol. Dial. Transplant, 4,* 40-44.

[12] Boim, M. A., dos Santos, O. F., Barros, E. J. & Schor, N. (1997). Glomerular hemodynamics in acute renal failure. *Ren. Fail, 19,* 209-212.

[13] Camussi, G., Ronco, C., Montrucchio, G. & Piccoli, G. (1998). Role of soluble mediators in sepsis and renal failure. *Kidney Int., 53,* S66, S38–S42.

[14] Casey, L. C. B. R. & Bone, R. C. (1993). Plasma cytokine and endotoxin levels correlate with survival in patients with the sepsis syndrome. *Ann. Intern. Med, 119,* 771–778.

[15] Pinsky, M. R. V. J., Deviere, J., Alegre, M., Kahn, R. J. & Dupont, E. (1993) Serum cytokine levels in human septic shock. Relation to multiple-system organ failure and mortality. *Chest, 103*, 565–575.

[16] Bone, R. C. & Newton, I. (1996). SEPSIS, SIRS, and CARS. *Crit. Care. Med., 24*, 1125–1128.

[17] Jaber, B. L. & Pereira, B. J. G. (1996). Inflammatory mediators in sepsis: rationale for extracorporeal therapies. *Am. J. Kidney Dis., 28*, S35–S49.

[18] Thijs, A. & Thijs, L. G. (1998). Pathogenesis of renal failure in sepsis. *Kidney Int., 66*, S34–S37.

[19] Uddman, E., Moller, S., Adner, M. & Edvinsson, L. (1999). Cytokines induce increased endothelin ET(B) receptor-mediated contraction. *Eur. J. Pharmacol, 376*, 223–232.

[20] Tschaikowsky, K., Sagner, S., Lehnert, N., Kaul, M. & Ritter, J. (2000). Endothelin in septic patients: effects on cardiovascular and renal function and its relationship to proinflammatory cytokines. *Crit. Care. Med, 28*, 1854–1860.

[21] Flo, T. H., Halaas, O., Torp, S., Ryan, L., Lien, E., Dybdahl, B., Sundan, A. & Espevik, T. (2001). Differential expression of Toll-like receptor 2 in human cells. *J. Leukoc. Biol, 69*, 474-481.

[22] Cunningham, P. N., Dyanov, H. M., Park, P., Wang, J., Newell, K. A. & Quigg, R. J. (2002). Acute renal failure in endotoxemia is caused by TNF acting directly on TNF receptor-1 in kidney. *J. Immun, 168*, 5817-5823.

[23] Bonventre, J. V. & Weinberg, J. M. (2003). Recent advances in the pathophysiology of ischemic acute renal failure. *J. Am. Soc. Nephrol, 14*, 2199-210.

[24] Linas, S. L., Whittenburg, D., Parsons, P. E. & Repine, J. E. (1992). Mild renal ischemia activates primed neutrophils to cause acute renal failure. *Kidney Int, 42*, 610-616.

[25] Bernard, G. R., Vincent, J. L. & Laterre, P. F. (2001). Efficacy and safety of recombinant human activated protein C for severe sepsis. *N. Engl. J. Med, 344*, 699-709.

[26] Jaber, B. L., Madhumathi, R., Daqing, G., Vaidyanathapuram, S., Perianayagam, M. C., Freeman, R. B. & Pereira, B. J. (2004). Cytokine gene promoter polymorphisms and mortality in acute renal failure. *Cytokine, 25*, 212-219.

[27] Fekete, A., Treszl, A., Toth-Heyn, P., Vannay, A., Tordai, A., Tulassay, T. & Vasarhelyi, B. (2003). Association between heat shock protein 72 gene polymorphism and acute renal failure in premature neonates. *Pediatr. Res, 54*, 452-455.

[28] Vicencio, A., Bidmon, B., Ryu, J., Reidy, K., Thulin, G., Mann, A., Gaudio, K. M., Kashgarian, M. & Siegel, N. J. (2003). Developmental expression of HSP-72 and ischemic tolerance of the immature kidney. *Pediatr. Nephrol, 18*, 85–91.

[29] Vasarhelyi, B., Toth-Heyn, P., Treszl, A. & Tulassay, T. (2005). Genetic polymorphisms and risk for acute renal failure in preterm neonates. *Pediatr. Nephrol., 20*, 132-135.

[30] Stuber, F., Petersen, M., Bokelmann, F. & Schade, U. (1996). A genomic polymorphism within the tumor necrosis factor locus influences plasma tumor necrosis factor-β concentrations and outcome of patients with severe sepsis. *Crit. Care. Med, 24*, 381-384.

[31] Fang, X. M., Schroder, S., Hoeft, A. & Stuber, F. (1999). Comparison of two polymorphisms of the interleukin-1 gene family: interleukin-1 receptor antagonist

polymorphism contributes to susceptibility to severe sepsis. *Crit. Care. Med, 27*, 1330-1334.

[32] Treszl, A., Toth-Heyn, P., Kocsis, I., Nobilis, A., Schuler, A., Tulassay, T. & Vasarhelyi, B. (2002). Interleukin genetic variants and the risk of renal failure in infants with infection. *Pediatr. Nephrol, 17*, 713-717.

[33] Lowe, P. R., Galley, H. F., Abdel-Fattah, A. & Webster, N. R. (2003). Influence of interleukin-10 polymorphisms on interleukin-10 expression and survival in critically ill patients. *Crit. Care. Med, 31*, 34-38.

[34] Gibot, S., Cariou, A., Drouet, L., Rossignol, M. & Ripoll, L. (2002). Association between a genomic polymorphism within the CD14 locus and septic shock susceptibility and mortality rate. *Crit. Care Med, 30*, 969-973.

[35] Waterer, G. W., ElBahlawan, L., Quasney, M. W., Zhang, Q., Kessler, L. A. & Wunderink, R. G. (2003). Heat shock protein 70-2+1267 AA homozygotes have an increased risk of septic shock in adults with community-acquired pneumonia. *Crit. Care. Med, 31*, 1367-1372.

[36] Child, N. J., Yang, I. A., Pulletz, M. C., de Courcy-Golder, K., Andrews, A. L., Pappachan, V. J. & Holloway, J. W. (2003). Polymorphisms in Toll-like receptor 4 and the systemic inflammatory response syndrome. *Biochem. Soc. Trans, 31*, 652-3.

[37] Ader, R., Cohen, N. & Felten, D. (1995). Psychoneuroimmunology: interactions between the nervous system and the immune system. *Lancet, 345*, 99–103.

[38] Bergquist, J., Tarkowski, A., Ekman, R. & Ewing, A. (1994). Discovery of endogenous catecholamines in lymphocytes and evidence for catecholamine regulation of lymphocyte function via an autocrine loop. *Proc. Natl. Acad. Sci. U. S. A., 91*, 12912–12916.

[39] Josefsson, E., Bergquist, J., Ekman, R. & Tarkowski, A. (1996). Catecholamines are synthesized by mouse lymphocytes and regulate function of these cells by induction of apoptosis. *Immunology, 88*, 140–146.

[40] Sanders, V. M., Baker, R. A., Ramer-Quinn, D. S., Kasprowicz, D. J., Fuchs, B. A. & Street, N. E. (1997). Differential expression of the β₂-adrenergic receptor by Th1 and Th2 clones: implications for cytokine production and B cell help. *J. Immunol, 158*, 4200–4210.

[41] Gaballa, M. A., Peppel, K., Lefkowitz, R. J., Aguirre, M., Dolber, P. C., Pennock, G. D., Koch, W. J. & Goldman, S. (1998). Enhanced vasorelaxation by overexpression of β₂-adrenergic receptors in large arteries. *J. Mol Cell Cardiol, 30*, 1037–1045.

[42] Chruscinski, A. J., Rohrer, D. K., Schauble, E., Desai, K. H., Bernstein, D. & Kobilka, B. K. (1999). Targeted disruption of the β₂ adrenergic receptor gene. *J. Biol. Chem., 274*, 16694–16700.

[43] Iaccarino, G., Cipolletta, E., Fiorillo, A., Annecchiarico, M., Ciccarelli, M., Cimini, V., Koch, W. J. & Trimarco, B. (2002). β₂-adrenergic receptor gene delivery to the endothelium corrects impaired adrenergic vasorelaxation in hypertension. *Circulation, 106*, 349-355.

[44] Nakamura, A., Niimi, R. & Yanagawa, Y. (2007). Renal effects of β₂-adrenoceptor agonist and clinical analysis in children. *Pediatr Res, 61*, 129-133.

[45] Nakamura, A., Imaizumi, A., Kohsaka, T., Yanagawa, Y. & Johns, E. J. (2000). β_2-adrenoceptor agonist suppresses tumour necrosis factor production in rat mesangial cells. *Cytokine, 12*, 491-494.

[46] Liao, J., Keiser, J. A., Scales, W. E., Kunkel, S. L. & Kluger, M. J. (1995). Role of epinephrine in TNF and IL-6 production from isolated perfused rat liver. *Am. J. Physiol, 268*, R896-R901.

[47] Severn, A., Rapson, N. T., Hunter, C. A. & Liew, F. Y. (1992). Regulation of tumor necrosis factor production by adrenaline and β-adrenergic agonists. *J. Immunol, 148*, 3441-3445.

[48] Hetier, P., Ayala, J., Bousseau, A. & Prochiantz, A. (1991). Modulation of interleukin-1 and tumor necrosis factor expression by β-adrenergic agonists in mouse ameboid microgial cells. *Exp. Brain Res, 86*, 407-413.

[49] Bernardin, G., Strosberg, A. D., Bernard, A., Mattei, M. & Marullo, S. (1998). Beta-adrenergic receptor-dependent and -independent stimulation of adenylate cyclase is impaired during severe sepsis in humans. *Intensive Care Med, 24*, 1315-1322

[50] Schmidt, W., Hacker, A., Gebhard, M. M., Martin, E. & Schmidt, H. (1998). Dopexamine attenuates endotoxin-induced microcirculatory changes in rat mesentery: role of β_2 adrenoceptors. *Crit. Care. Med, 26,* 1639-1645.

[51] Tighe, D., Moss, R. & Bennett, D. (1996). Cell surface adrenergic receptor stimulation modifies the endothelial response to SIRS. Systemic Inflammatory Response Syndrome. *New Horiz, 4*, 426-442.

[52] Tighe, D., Moss, R. & Bennett, D. (1998). Porcine hepatic response to sepsis and its amplification by an adrenergic receptor alpha1 agonist and a β_2 antagonist. *Clin. Sci (Lond)., 95*, 467-478.

[53] Sigurdsson, G. H., Christenson, J. T., al-Mousawi, M. & Owunwanne, A. (1989). Use of indium-111 oxine to study pulmonary and hepatic leukocyte sequestration in endotoxin shock and effects of the β_2 receptor agonist terbutaline. *Am. J. Physiol Imaging, 4*, 136-142.

[54] Nakamura, A. & Yanagawa, Y. (2008). Pharmacogenomics and sepsis-induced renal failure: Effects of β_2-adrenoceptor function on the course of sepsis. *Current Pharmacogenomics and Personalized Medicine, 6*, 98-107.

[55] Nakamura, A., Imaizumi, A., Yanagawa, Y., Niimi, R. & Kohsaka, T. (2003). Suppression of tumor necrosis factor-alpha by β_2-adrenoceptor activation: role of mitogen-activated protein kinases in renal mesangial cells. *Inflammation Res., 52*, 26-31.

[56] Nakamura, A., Johns, E. J., Imaizumi, A., Yanagawa, Y. & Kohsaka, T. (1999). Effect of β_2-adrenoceptor activation and angiotensin II on tumour necrosis factor and interleukin-6 genes transcription in the rat renal resident macrophage cells. *Cytokine, 11*, 759–65.

[57] Weiss, M., Schneider, E. M., Tarnow, J. Mettler, S. Krone, M. Teschemacher, A, & Lemoine H. (1996). Is inhibition of oxygen radical production of neutrophils by sympathomimetics mediated via β_2 adrenoceptors? *J. Pharmacol Exp. Ther, 278,* 1105-1113.

[58] Svensjo, E., Persson, C. G. & Rutili, G. (1977). Inhibition of bradykinin-induced macromolecular leakage from postcapillary venules by a β₂-AR stimulant, terbutaline. *Acta. Physiol. Scand, 101*, 504-506.

[59] Makhlouf, K., Comabella, M., Imitola, J., Weiner, H. L. & Khoury, S. J. (2001). Oral salbutamol decreases IL-12 in patients with secondary progressive multiple sclerosis. *J. Neuroimmunol, 117*, 156–165.

[60] Malfait, A. M., Malik, A. S., Marinova-Mutafchieva, L., Butler, D. M., Maini, R. N. & Feldmann, M. (1999). The β₂-adrenergic agonist salbutamol is a potent suppressor of established collagen-induced arthritis: mechanisms of action. *J. Immunol, 162*, 6278–6283.

[61] Tiegs, G., Bang, R. & Neuhuber, W. L. (1999). Requirement of peptidergic sensory innervation for disease activity in murine models of immune hepatitis and protection by β-adrenergic stimulation. *J. Neuroimmunol, 96*, 131–143.

[62] Van der Poll, T., Coyle, S. M., Barbosa, K., Braxton, C. C. & Lowry, S. F. (1996). Epinephrine inhibits tumor necrosis factor-β and potentiates interleukin-10 production during human endotoxemia. *J. Clin. Invest, 97*, 713-719.

[63] Van der Pouw-Kraan, T. C. T. M., Boeije, L. C. M., Smeenk, R. J. T., Wijdenes, J. & Aarden, L. A. (1995). Prostaglandin-E₂ is a potent inhibitor of human interleukin 12 production. *J. Exp. Med, 181*, 775-779.

[64] Strassmann, G., Patil-Koota, V., Finkelman, F., Fong, M. & Kambayashi, T. (1994). Evidence for the involvement of interleukin 10 in the differential deactivation of murine peritoneal macrophages by prostaglandin E₂. *J. Exp. Med., 180*, 2365-2370.

[65] Panina-Bordignon, P. J., Mazzeo, D., Di Lucia, P. D'Ambrosio, D. Lang, R. Fabbri, L. Self, C. & Sinigaglia, F. (1997). β₂-agonists prevent Th1 development by selective inhibition of interleukin 12. *J. Clin. Invest, 100*, 1513–1519.

[66] Koepke, J. P. & Dibona, G. F. (1986). Central adrenergic receptor control of renal function in conscious hypertensive rats. *Hypertension, 8,* 133–141.

[67] Shimkets, R. A., Warnock, D. G., Bositis, C. M., Nelson-Williams, C., Hansson, J. H., Schambelan, M. Gill, Jr. Ulick, S. Milora, R. V. & Findling, J. W. (1994). Liddle's syndrome: heritable human hypertension caused by mutations in the β subunit of the epithelial sodium channel. *Cell, 79*, 407–414.

[68] DiBona, G. F. & Kopp, U. C. (1997). Neural control of renal function. *Physiol. Rev., 77*, 75–197.

[69] Boivin, V., Jahns, R., Gambaryan, S., Ness, W., Boege, F. & Lohse, M. J. (2001). Immunofluorescent imaging of β₁- and β₂-adrenergic receptors in rat kidney. *Kidney Int., 59,* 515-531.

[70] Pradervand, S., Barker, P. M., Wang, Q. & Ernst, S. A. (1999). Beermann F., Grubb B. R., Burnier M., Schmidt A., Bindels R. J., Gatzy J. T., Rossier B. C., Hummler E. Salt restriction induces pseudohypoaldosteronism type 1 in mice expressing low levels of the β-subunit of the amiloride-sensitive epithelial sodium channel. *Proc. Natl. Acad. Sci. U. S. A., 96,* 1732–1737.

[71] Snyder, P. M. (2000). Liddle's syndrome mutations disrupt cAMP-mediated translocation of the epithelial Na⁺ channel to the cell surface. *J. Clin. Invest, 105*, 45–53.

[72] Wallace, D. P., Reif, G., Hedge, A. M., Thrasher, J. B. & Pietrow, P. (2004). Adrenergic regulation of salt and fluid secretion in human medullary collecting duct cells. *Am. J. Physiol. Renal Physiol, 287,* F639–F648.

[73] Tago, K. & Schuster, V. L. & Stokes, J. B. (1986). Regulation of chloride self exchange by cAMP in cortical collecting tubule. *Am. J. Physiol, 251,* F40-48.

[74] Singh, H. & Linas, S. (1997). Role of protein kinase C in β_2-adrenoceptor function in cultured rat proximal tubular epithelial cells. *Am. J. Physiol, 273,* F193-F199.

[75] Hashimoto, K., Shintani, S., Yamashita, S., Tei, S., Takai, M., Tsutsui, M., Kawamura, K., Ohkawa, T., Hiyama, T. & Yabuuchi, Y. (1979). Pharmacological properties of procaterol, a newly synthetized, specific β_2-adrenoceptor stimulant. Part II. Effects on the peripheral organs (author's transl). *Nippon Yakurigaku Zasshi, 75,* 333-364. (Japanese).

[76] Main, I. W., Nikolic-paterson, D. J. & Atkins, R. C. (1992). T cells and macrophages and their role in renal injury. *Semin Nephrol, 12,* 395-407.

[77] Klahr, S. (1993). Interstitial macrophages. *Semin Nephrol, 13,* 388-395.

[78] Fougueray, B., Philipp, C., Herbelin, A. & Perez, J., Ardaillov, R. & Baud, L. (1993). Cytokine formation within rat glomeruli during experimental endotoxaemia. *J. Am. Soc. Nephrol, 3,* 1783-1791.

[79] Kayama, E., Yoshida, T., Kodama, Y., Matsui, T., Matheson, J. M. & Luster, M. I. (1997). Proinflammatory cytokines and interleukin-6 in the renal response to bacterial endotoxin. *Cytokine, 9,* 688-695.

[80] Nakamura. A., Johns, E. J., Imaizumi, A., Yanagawa, Y. & Kohsaka, T. (1999). Modulation of interleukin-6 by β_2-adrenoceptor in endotoxin-stimulated renal macrophage. *Kidney Int., 56,* 839-849.

[81] Hirano, T. & Kishimoto, T. (1990). Interleukin-6. In *Handbook of Experimental Pharmacology, (95)* edited by Sporn MB, Roberts AB, Berlin, Springer-Verlag, 633-665.

[82] Maimone, D. C., Cioni, C., Rosa, S., Machia, G., Aloisi, F. & Annunziata, P. (1993). Norepinephrine and vasoactive intestinal peptide induce interleukin-6 secretion by astrocytes. *J. Neuroimmunol, 47,* 73-81.

[83] Zhang, Y., Lin, Jian-Xin. J. & Vilcek, J. (1988). Synthesis of interleukin-6 in human fibroblasts is triggered by increase in intracellular cyclic AMP. *J. Biol. Chem., 263,* 6177-6182.

[84] Straub, R. H., Hermann, M., Frauenholz, T., Berkmiller, G., Lang, B., Scholmerich, J and Falk, W. (1996). Neuroimmune control of interleukin-6 secretion in the murine spleen. *J. Neuroimmunol, 71,* 37-43

[85] Nakamura, A., Johns, E. J., Imaizumi, A., Abe, T. & Kohsaka, T. (1998). Regulation of tumour necrosis factor and interleukin-6 gene transcription by beta2-adrenoceptor in the rat astrocytes. *J. Neuroimmunol, 88,* 144-153.

[86] Kaplan, B. S., Meyers, K. E. & Schulman, S. L. (1998). The pathogeneis and treatment of hemolytic uremic syndrome. *J. Am. Soc. Nephrol, 8,* 1126-1133.

[87] Fong, J. S., De Chadarevian, J. P. & Kaplan, B. S. (1982). Hemolytic Uremic Syndrome. Current concepts and management. *Pediatr. Clin. N. Am., 29,* pp. 835–856.

[88] Van De Kar, N. C., Monnens, L. A., Karmali, M. A. & Van Hinsbergh, V. W. (1992). Tumour necrosis factor and interleukin-1 induce expression of the verocytotoxin

receptor globotriaosylceramide on human vascular endothelial cells: Implications for the pathogenesis of the hemolytic uremic syndrome. *Blood, 80,* 2755-2764.

[89] Lingwood, C. A. (1994). Verotoxin-binding in human renal sections. *Nephron, 66,* 21 – 28.

[90] Kiyokawa, N., Taguchi, T., Mori, T., Uchida, H., Sato, N., Takeda, T. & Fujimoto, J. (1998). Induction of apoptosis in normal human renal tubular epithelial cells by Escherichia coli shiga toxin 1 and 2. *J. Infect Dis., 178,* 178-184.

[91] Hughes, A. K., Stricklett, P. K. & Kohan, D. E. (1998). Cytotoxic effect of shiga toxin-1 on human proximal tubule cells. *Kidney Int., 54,* 426-437.

[92] Zhu, Y., Prehn, J. H. M., Culmsee, C. & Krieglstein, J. (1999). The β₂-adrenoceptor agonist clenbuterol modulates Bcl-2, Bcl-xl and Bax protein expression following transient forebrain ischemia. *Neuroscience, 90,* 1255-1263.

[93] Nakamura, A., Imaizumi, A., Yanagawa, Y., Niimi, R., Kohsaka, T. & Johns, E. J. (2003). β₂-adrenoceptor activation inhibits Shiga toxin2-induced apoptosis of renal tubular epithelial cells. *Biochem Pharmacol, 66,* 343-53.

[94] Beutler, B. (2000). TRL4: central component of the sole mammalian LPS sensor. *Curr Opin Immunol, 12,* 20-6.

[95] Poltorak, A., He, X., Smirnova, I., Liu, M. Y., Van Huffel, C., Du, X. Birdwell, D. Alejos, E. Silva, M. Galanos, C. Freudenberg, M. Ricciardi-Castagnoli, P. Layton, B. & Beutler, B. (1998). Defective LPS signaling in C3H/HeJ and C57BL/10ScCr mice: mutations in Tlr4 gene. *Science, 282,* 2085-8.

[96] Chen, G., Li, J., Ochani, M., Rendon-Mitchell, B., Qiang, X., Susarla, S., Ulloa, L.,Yang, H., Fan, S., Goyert, S. M., Wang, P., Tracey, K. J., Sama, A. E., and Wang, H. (2004). Bacterial endotoxin stimulates macrophages to release HMGB1 partly through CD14- and TNF-dependent mechanisms. *J. Leukoc Biol, 76,* 994-1001.

[97] Cunningham, P. N., Wang, Y., Guo, R., He, G. & Quigg, R. J. (2004). Role of Toll-like receptor 4 in endotoxin-induced acute renal failure. *J. Immunol, 172,* 2629-35.

[98] Nakamura, A., Niimi, R. & Yanagawa, Y. (2009). Renal β₂-adrenoceptor modulates the lipopolysaccharide transport system in sepsis-induced acute renal failure. *Inflammation, 32,*12-19.

[99] Nakamura, A., Johns, E. J., Imaizumi, A., Yanagawa, Y. & Kohsaka, T. (1997). β₂-adrenoceptor activation and angiotensin II regulate tumour necrosis factor and interleukin-6 genes transcription in the rat renal resident macrophage and mesangial cells. *J. Am. Soc. Nephrol, 8,* 479A (abstract)

[100] Nakamura, A., Johns, E. J., Imaizumi, A., Yanagawa, Y. & Kohsaka, T. (2000). β₂-adrenoceptor agonist suppresses renal tumour necrosis factor and enhances interleukin-6 gene expression induced by endotoxin. *Nephrol Dial Transplant., 15,* 1928-1934.

[101] Richardson, S. E., Karmali, M. A., Becker, L. E. & Smith, C. R. (1988). The histopathology of the hemolytic uremic syndrome associated with verocytotoxin-producing Escherichia coli infection. *Human Pathol, 19 ,* 1102-1108.

[102] Inward, C., Howie, A., Fitspatrick, M., Rafaat, F., Milford, D. & Taylor, C. M. (1997). Renal histopathology in fetal cases of diarrhea-associated hemolytic uremic syndrome. British Association of Paediatric Nephrology. *Pediatr Nephrol, 11,* 556 –559.

[103] Taguchi, T., Uchida, H., Kiyokawa, N., Mori, T., Sato, N., Horie, H., Takeda, T. & Fujimoto, J. (1998). Verotoxins induce apoptosis in human renal tubular epithelium derived cells. *Kidney Int., 53,* 1681 –1688.

[104] Emilien, G. & Maloteaux, J. M. (1998). Current therapeutic uses and potential of beta-adrenoceptor agonists and antagonists. *Eur J. Clin. Pharmacol, 53,* 389–404.

[105] Maurice, L. P., Hata, J. A., Shah, A. S., White, D. C., McDonald, P. H., Dolber, P. C., Wilson, K. H., Lefkowitz, R. J., Glower, D. D. & Koch, W. J. (1999). Enhancement of cardiac function after adenoviral-mediated in vivo intracoronary 2-adrenergic receptor gene delivery. *J. Clin. Invest ,104,* 21–29.

[106] Begany, D. P., Carcillo, J. A., Herzer, W. A., Mi, Z. & Jackson, E. K. (1996). Inhibition of type IV phosphodiesterase by Ro 20-1724 attenuates endotoxin-induced acute renal failure. *J. Pharmacol Exp. Ther., 278,* 37-41.

[107] Guan, Z., Miller, S. B. & Greenwald, J. E. (1995). Zaprinast accelerates recovery from established acute renal failure in the rat. *Kidney Int., 47,* 1569–1575.

[108] Huard, J., Lochmuller, H., Acsadi, G., Jani, A., Massie, B. & Karpati, G. (1995). The route of administration is a major determinant of the transduction efficiency of rat tissues by adenoviral recombinants. *Gene Ther., 2,* 107–115

[109] Chuah, M. K., Collen, D. & Vanden Driessche, T. (2003). Biosafety of adenoviral vectors. Curr. *Gene Ther., 3,* 527–543

[110] Nakamura, A., Imaizumi, A., Yanagawa, Y., Niimi, R., Kohsaka, T. & Johns, E. J. (2005). Adenoviral delivery of the beta$_2$-adrenoceptor gene in sepsis. *Clin. Science, 109,* 503-511.

[111] Elkon, K. B., Liu, C. C., Gall, J. G. Trevejo, J., Marino, M. W., Abrahamsen, K. A., Song, X., Zhou, J. L., Old, L. J., Crystal, R. G., and Falck-Pedersen, E. (1997) . TNF-α plays a central role in immune-mediated clearance of adenoviral vectors. *Proc. Natl. Acad. Sci. U. S. A., 94,* 9814–9819 .

[112] Zhang, H. G., Zhou, T., Yang, C., Edwards, P. K., Curiel, D. T. & Mountz, J. D. (1998). Inhibition of TNF-α decreases inflammation and prolongs adenovirus gene expression in lung and liver. Hum. *Gene Ther., 9,* 1875–1884.

[113] Alexander, S., Bramson, J., Foley, R. & Xing, Z. (2004). Protection from endotoxemia by adenoviral-mediated gene transfer of human bactericidal/permeability-increasing protein. *Blood, 103,* 93–99.

[114] Minter, R. M., Ferry, M. A., Murday, M. E. Tannahill, C. L., Bahjat, F. R., Oberholzer, C., Oberholzer, A., LaFace, D., Hutchins, B., Wen, S., Shinoda, J., Copeland, E. M. 3rd, and Moldawer, L. L. (2001). Adenoviral delivery of human and viral IL-10 in murine sepsis. *J. Immunol., 167,* 1053–1059.

[115] Sparrow, A. & Willis, F. (2004). Management of septic shock in childhood. Emerg. Med. *Australasia, 16,* 125–134.

In: Acute Kidney Injury: Causes, Diagnosis and Treatments   ISBN: 978-1-61209-790-9
Editor: Jonathan D. Mendoza, pp. 167-171   © 2011 Nova Science Publishers, Inc.

Short Communication

Role of Oxidative Stress in Renal Ischemia/Reperfusion Injury

Satoshi Hagiwara[*], *Hironori Koga and Takayuki Noguchi*

Oita University Faculty of Medicine, Department of Anesthesiology and Intensive Care
Medicine, 1-1 Idaigaoka Hasama-machi, Yufu City, Oita, 879-5593, Japan

Abstract

Acute kidney injury (AKI) occurs frequently in various clinical contexts. There is increasing evidence that AKI directly contributes to dysfunction in the lung, brain, liver, heart, and other organs. Various drugs have been developed and are now being used clinically, but with limited success. AKI continues to contribute significantly to morbidity and mortality in the intensive care unit (ICU) setting, especially when associated with distant organ dysfunction. Recently, many studies have examined the mechanisms underlying AKI. In particular, the role of reactive oxygen species (ROS) in AKI pathogenesis has received much attention. ROS include hydroxyl radicals that react with nearby tissues, proteins, enzymes, cell membranes, and DNA. Hydroxyl radicals themselves are short-lived, but they damage biomolecules, affecting cellular and tissue function. The key location for ROS generation is the mitochondrion. Excessive ROS generation damages the mitochondria themselves, leading to cellular dysfunction and apoptosis. Anti-oxidants are involved in regulating intracellular ROS levels and are generally thought to attenuate oxidative stress, cellular and tissue injury, and mitochondrial damage. These findings collectively point to ROS as important targets for AKI treatment.

[*] Tel: +81-97-586-5943, Fax:+81-97-586-5949, E-mail:saku@oita-u.ac.jp

Epidemiology of Acute Kidney Injury

Acute kidney injury (AKI) can result from a variety of conditions and has serious consequences. Indeed, AKI occurs in 1% of hospital admissions and up to 7% of hospitalized patients develop AKI [1]. AKI occurs commonly in the intensive care unit (ICU); about 25% of ICU patients develop AKI and 5% of patients in the ICU will need renal replacement therapy [1]. AKI can also cause serious problems in other organs. The mortality rate in AKI patients remains high despite significant advances in medical care [2-4]. AKI is considered a life-limiting disease.

Mechanisms of Acute Kidney Injury

In recent studies, several mechanisms of AKI have been examined. In AKI, renal endothelial cells and proximal tubular epithelial cells produce cytokines and chemokines that result in infiltration of inflammatory cells into the interstitium of the kidney [5]. Inflammatory cells in the kidney also produce pro- and anti-inflammatory cytokines that can further increase inflammation, leading to kidney dysfunction [5]. Adherent and infiltrating leukocytes can cause tubular epithelial and endothelial injury by releasing potent vasoconstrictors, including prostaglandins, leukotrienes, and thromboxanes [6], as well as direct endothelial injury by releasing endothelin and decreasing nitric oxide (NO) [7, 8]. Thus, the main causes of AKI can be summarized as endothelial injury from vascular perturbations, direct effects of nephrotoxins, abolition of renal autoregulation, and the formation of inflammatory mediators.

Reactive Oxygen Species and Acute Kidney Injury

A recent study indicated that mitochondrial damage is a key contributor to renal tubular cell death in AKI [9]. Mitochondrial dysfunction can be caused by various mechanisms. One involves reactive oxygen species (ROS; Figure 1). ROS originate from several sources, including NADPH, xanthine oxidase-hypoxanthine, inflammatory cells, and the mitochondria of parenchymal cells, due to cell dysfunction-provoked derangement of the electron transport chain.

ROS are produced in the normal processes of cell metabolism, and cells possess several ROS-scavenging and -detoxifying systems. However, *excessive* ROS can be produced in inflammation, infection, and ischemia/reperfusion (Figure 1, 2). ROS in quiescent mitochondria pose a risk to the organelle and cell viability through the opening of mitochondrial membrane channels, including mitochondrial permeability transition pores (mPTPs) and inner membrane anion channels, leading to a collapse in mitochondrial membrane potential and further transient increases in ROS generation from the electron transport chain. These events may result in autophagy, apoptosis, or necrosis [10, 11]. Excessive ROS also damage proteins, lipids, and DNA, and further stimulate aspects of the inflammatory response [12, 13].

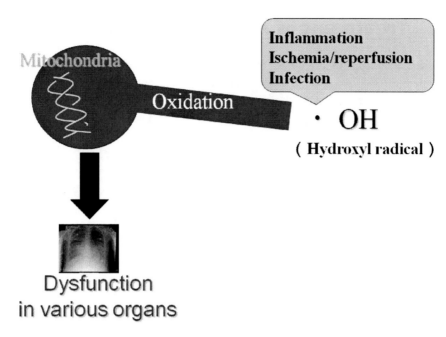

Figure 1. Relationship between mitochondria and ROS.

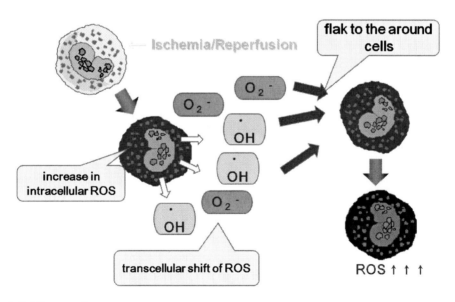

Figure 2. ROS generation.

ROS are induced in various types of AKI and can cause renal tubule cell injury by protein oxidation, lipid peroxidation, and DNA damage, leading to apoptosis [14]. Increased ROS generation has been shown to affect cell function and structure, enzyme function, transcription, and vascular and endothelial function, in particular, through mitochondrial dysfunction [15]. Consistent with the roles of ROS, we previously demonstrated that ETS-GS, a new anti-oxidative drug, significantly improves AKI [16]. ROS and their effects are now considered major issues in the pathophysiology of AKI.

Treatment of AKI: Present and Future

After a diagnosis of AKI and therapeutic options have been exhausted, the clinical management of AKI becomes primarily supportive, with renal replacement therapy (RRT) as the central component of care for patients with severe AKI. Generally accepted indications for RRT include volume overload, hyperkalemia, metabolic acidosis, and overt uremic symptoms.

Several drugs, such as insulin-like growth factor 1, thyroxine, atrial natriuretic peptide, low-dose dopamine, and loop diuretics, have been used in patients with AKI. Unlike some of the more recent drugs, the use of loop diuretics in AKI has persisted despite a lack of evidence that they confer any real benefit, such as decreased mortality or renal recovery [17-21].

Given the failure of many drugs in AKI therapy, novel agents are needed, with efficacy demonstrated in well-designed clinical trials. Anti-oxidative drugs, such as ETS-GS, are promising and have shown favorable results in preclinical studies. Other investigational compounds are being examined in clinical trials for a variety of indications. When possible, we have indicated whether anti-oxidative drugs, such as ETS-GS, are in human studies for other indications; information from such studies may facilitate clinical trials for their use in AKI.

Conclusions

AKI is a common disease in the ICU. Several new treatment methods have been developed, including renal replacement therapy. Several drugs have demonstrated efficacy in preventing or ameliorating experimental AKI [22], but none of these have been clinically successful. Thus, there is a continuing need for new drugs to treat AKI. Recent studies have indicated that anti-oxidative drugs may be useful in the treatment of AKI.

References

[1]   Lameire N, Van Biesen W, Vanholder R. The changing epidemiology of acute renal failure. *Nature Clinical Practice Nephrology*. 2006;2(7):364–377.

[2]   Uchino S, Bellomo R, Goldsmith D, Bates S, Ronco C. An assessment of the RIFLE criteria for acute renal failure in hospitalized patients. *Crit. Care Med.* 2006;34:1913–1917.

[3]   Hoste EA, Clermont G, Kersten A, et al. RIFLE criteria for acute kidney injury are associated with hospital mortality in critically ill patients: a cohort analysis. *Crit. Care.* 2006;10:R73.

[4]   Uchino S, Kellum JA, Bellomo R, et al. Acute renal failure in critically ill patients: a multinational, multicenter study. *JAMA*. 2005;294:813–818.

[5]   Kinsey GR, Li L, Okusa MD. Inflammation in acute kidney injury. *Nephron Exp Nephrol.* 2008;109(4):e102-7.

[6]   Klausner JM, Paterson IS, Goldman G, et al. Postischemic renal injury is mediated by neutrophils and leukotrienes. *American Journal of Physiology.* 1989;256(5):F794–F802.

[7]   Linas S, Whittenburg D, Repine JE. Nitric oxide prevents neutrophil-mediated acute renal failure. *American Journal of Physiology.* 1997;272(1):F48–F54.

[8]   Caramelo C, Espinosa G, Manzarbeitia F, et al. Role of endothelium-related mechanisms in the pathophysiology of renal ischemia/reperfusion in normal rabbits. *Circulation Research.* 1996;79(5):1031–1038.

[9]   Bonventre J.V., Weinberg J.M. Recent advances in the pathophysiology of ischemic acute renal failure. *J. Am. Soc. Nephrol.* 2003;14:2199–2210.

[10]   Lemasters JJ, Nieminen AL, Qian T, Trost LC, Elmore SP, Nishimura Y, Crowe RA, Cascio WE, Bradham CA, Brenner DA, Herman B. The mitochondrial permeability transition in cell death: a common mechanism in necrosis, apoptosis and autophagy. *Biochim. Biophys. Acta.* 1998;1366:177–196.

[11]   Wang W, Fang H, Groom L, Cheng A, Zhang W, Liu J, Wang X, Li K, Han P, Zheng M, Yin J, Mattson MP, Kao JP, Lakatta EG, Sheu SS, Ouyang K, Chen J, Dirksen RT, Cheng H. Superoxide flashes in single mitochondria. *Cell.* 2008;134:279–290.

[12]   Lum H, Roebuck KA. Oxidant stress and endothelial cell dysfunction. *Am. J. Physiol. Cell Physiol.* 280: C719–C741, 2001.

[13]   Land W. Impact of the reperfusion injury on acute and chronic rejection events following clinical cadaveric renal transplantation. *Clin. Invest.* 72: 719, 1994.

[14]   Himmelfarb J, McMonagle E, Freedman S, Klenzak J, McMenamin E, Le P, Pupim LB, Ikizler TA; The PICARD Group: Oxidative stress is increased in critically ill patients with acute renal failure. *J. Am. Soc. Nephrol.* 15 : 2449–2456, 2004.

[15]   Lee H, Ha H, King G: Reactive Oxygen Species and Diabetic Nephropathy. *Am. Soc. of Nephr.* 2003; 14: S209-10.

[16]   Hagiwara S, Koga H, Iwasaka H, Kudo K, Hasegawa A, Kusaka J, Yokoi I, Noguchi T. ETS-GS, a New Antioxidant, Ameliorates Renal Ischemia-Reperfusion Injury in a Rodent Model. *J. Surg. Res.* 2010 [in press].

[17]   Miller SB, Martin DR, Kissane J, Hammerman MR. Insulin-like growth factor I accelerates recovery from ischemic acute tubular necrosis in the rat. *Proc. Natl. Acad. Sci. USA.* 1992;89:11876-11880.

[18]   Acker CG, Singh AR, Flick RP, Bernardini J, Greenberg A, Johnson JP. A trial of thyroxine in acute renal failure. *Kidney Int.* 2000;57:293 -298.

[19]   Rahman SN, Kim GE, Mathew AS, Goldberg CA, Allgren R, Schrier RW, et al. Effects of atrial natriuretic peptide in clinical acute renal failure. *Kidney Int.*1994; 45:1731 - 1738.

[20]   Chertow GM, Sayegh MH, Allgren RL, Lazarus JM. Is the administration of dopamine associated with adverse or favorable outcomes in acute renal failure? Auriculin Anaritide Acute Renal Failure Study Group. *Am. J. Med.*1996; 101:49 -53.

[21]   Conger JD. Interventions in clinical acute renal failure: what are the data? *Am. J. Kidney Dis.*1995; 26:565 -576.

[22]   Star RA. Treatment of acute renal failure. *Kidney Int.*1998; 54:1817 -1831

Index

D

M

S

T

U

V